Alzheimer's Disease

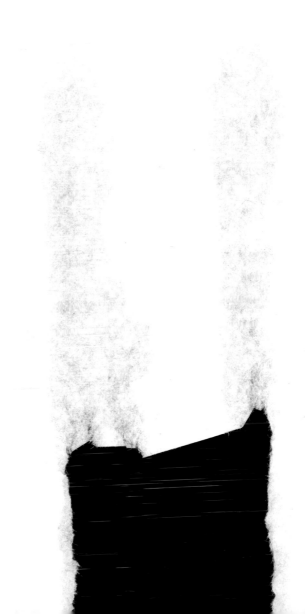

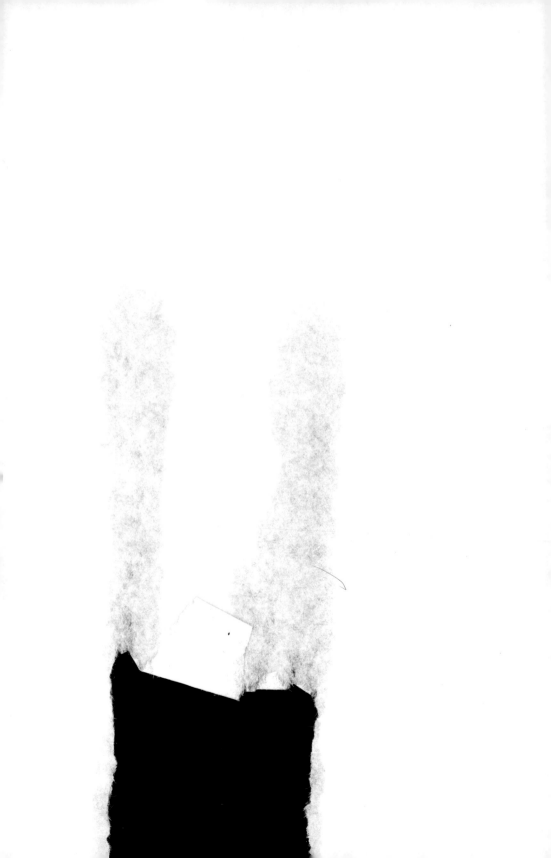

Alzheimer's Disease

PAUL DASH, MD
Assistant Clinical Professor of Neurology
LSU Health Sciences Center
New Orleans, Louisiana

AND

NICOLE VILLEMARETTE-PITTMAN, PhD
Research Coordinator, Epilepsy Center of Excellence
LSU Health Sciences Center
New Orleans, Louisiana

AUSTIN J. SUMNER, MD
Series Editor
Richard M. Paddison Professor and
Head, Department of Neurology
LSU Health Sciences Center
New Orleans, Louisiana

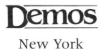

New York

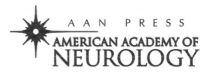

AAN PRESS
AMERICAN ACADEMY OF
NEUROLOGY

Demos Medical Publishing Inc., 368 Park Avenue South, New York, New York 10016

© 2005 by AAN Press, American Academy of Neurology, 1080 Montreal Avenue, Saint Paul, MN 55116. All rights reserved. This book is protected by copyright. No part of it may be reproduced, stored in a retrieval system, or transmitted in any form or by any means, electronic, mechanical, photocopying, recording, or otherwise, without prior written permission.

Uses for products within this text may include those not currently approved by the FDA. For more information on the products, please see full prescribing information.

Library of Congress Cataloging-in-Publication Data
Dash, Paul, 1954–
  Alzheimer's disease / Paul Dash and Nicole Villemarette-Pittman.
    p. cm.
  Includes index.
  ISBN 1-932603-12-3 (pbk. : alk. paper)
  1. Alzheimer's disease—Popular works. I. Villemarette-Pittman, Nicole, 1976–
II. Title.
  RC523.2.D37 2005
  616.8'31—dc22

                                                                2005005688

Printed in Canada

Contents

Dedication

To the caregivers—the true frontline warriors in the battle against Alzheimer's—you have our utmost respect and admiration for the incredible love and sacrifice you make on a daily basis for those suffering with dementia.

About the AAN Press Quality of Life Guides

IN THE SPIRIT OF THE DOCTOR-PATIENT PARTNERSHIP

THE BETTER-INFORMED PATIENT is often able to play a vital role in his or her own care. This is especially the case with neurologic disorders, for which effective management of disease can be promoted—indeed, *enhanced*—through patient education and involvement.

In the spirit of the partnership-in-care between physicians and patients, the American Academy of Neurology Press is pleased to produce a series of "Quality of Life" guides on an array of diseases and ailments that affect the brain and central nervous system. The series, produced in partnership with Demos Medical Publishing, answers a number of basic and important questions faced by patients and their families.

Additionally, the authors, most of whom are physicians and all of whom are experts in the areas in which they write, provide a detailed discussion of the disorder, its causes, and the course it may follow. You also find strategies for coping with the disorder and handling a number of nonmedical issues.

The result: As a reader, you will be able to develop a framework for understanding the disease and become better prepared to manage the life changes associated with it.

ABOUT THE AMERICAN ACADEMY OF NEUROLOGY (AAN)

The American Academy of Neurology is the premier organization for neurologists worldwide. In addition to support of educational and scientific advances, the AAN—along with its sister organization, the AAN Foundation—is a strong advocate of public education and a leading supporter of research for breakthroughs in neurologic patient care.

ix

More information on the activities of the AAN is available on our website, www.aan.com. For a better understanding of common disorders of the brain, as well as to learn about people living with these disorders, please turn to the AAN Foundation's website, www.thebrainmatters.org.

ABOUT NEUROLOGY AND NEUROLOGISTS

Neurology is the medical specialty associated with disorders of the brain and central nervous system. Neurologists are medical doctors with specialized training in the diagnosis, treatment, and management of patients suffering from neurologic disease.

Austin J. Sumner, M.D.
Series Editor, AAN Press Quality of Life Guides

Preface

WHILE ALL CULTURES RIGHTLY VALUE and respect the elderly for their wisdom and experience, older people may have problems with thinking and memory. The idea of senility has become synonymous with "getting old," and many people, including some doctors, anticipate that elderly people will lose a considerable degree of their mental prowess as a natural part of the aging process. This outdated perception is radically changing, and new evidence suggests that disabilities due to cognitive problems in the elderly are not a natural part of aging, but are, in fact, the result of disease processes, the most common cause being Alzheimer's disease.

As of 2003, an estimated 5 million Americans suffer from Alzheimer's disease, only half of whom have been diagnosed. An uncertain but even larger number have "mild cognitive impairment," often a precursor to Alzheimer's. By 2030, barring a cure for this illness, the number of individuals who will be diagnosed with Alzheimer's disease is estimated to be 8 million, and by 2050, 14 million. The cost in both suffering and dollars on the part of patients and families is enormous, and growing.

This book provides an overview of our current understanding of the causes, diagnosis, and treatment of Alzheimer's disease. It is designed to help caregivers and family members of people with Alzheimer's disease gain a better understanding of the nature of the disease process and the available options for coping with and managing this illness.

As a neurologist who has the privilege of working with Alzheimer's patients on a regular basis, I have drawn on my experiences with them and their families to present answers to many of the questions we typically encounter. Presenting information that is often highly technical in a way that people without medical training can understand is difficult. To this end, I enlisted the able assistance of my coauthor, Nicole Villemarette-Pittman. She helped to make the book more understandable and made significant contributions to the text that help convey the importance of education, preparation, and understanding in caring for an Alzheimer's patient.

We sincerely hope that you find this book both useful and informative. The subtitles of each chapter are written in question format to help readers search for the topics that most relate to their problems. A list of abbreviations and a glossary are provided at the end of the book. Italicized words in the text have glossary entries.

Paul Dash, M.D.

Acknowledgments

WE WERE BOTH HONORED and excited to take on the challenge of writing this book when invited to do so by Dr. Austin Sumner, editor-in-chief of the American Academy of Neurology's Quality of Life Guide series.

In addition to Dr. Sumner, we would like to thank Dr. Diana M. Schneider and her colleagues at Demos Medical Publishing for their skilled editorial assistance. We also thank our families for their patience and love in putting up with the seclusion we needed to research and write this book.

Finally, this book would not have been possible without the legions of scientist and physicians who have published many thousands of studies on Alzheimer's disease and dementia. Because this book was written for the general public, we have not cited the technical references for the studies mentioned in the text. To those who recognize their work being mentioned without formal attribution, we offer our esteem and our gratitude.

Alzheimer's Disease

Understanding Dementia and Alzheimer's Disease

Chapter Question:
Is there a difference between dementia and
Alzheimer's disease?

The term *dementia* is used to refer to a medical condition that involves the progressive loss of intellectual abilities. Although there are many types of dementia, Alzheimer's disease (AD) is by far the most common dementia. Chapter 1 discusses several definitions of dementia and AD in some detail.

A BRIEF HISTORY OF ALZHEIMER'S DISEASE

SCIENCE HAS COME a long way since 1907, when Dr. Alois Alzheimer first published a description of what he saw under the microscope when examining the brain of a patient who died of dementia in her 50s. At first, what is now known as AD was referred to as *presenile dementia*, a diagnosis reserved for patients under 60 to whom the more common illness of *senile dementia* did not seem to apply. Current convention does not distinguish presenile from senile dementia because there are no fundamental differences in disease pathology. As medicine has developed into an organized system of diagnoses based on behavioral, anatomic, and physiologic characteristics, so has AD developed into a dementia diagnosis with specific clinical presentations and biological markers.

DEFINITIONS OF DEMENTIA AND ALZHEIMER'S DISEASE

Although many people have a rudimentary understanding of the meaning of dementia, most are not aware of the potential causes or what key

> Alzheimer's disease is a form of dementia.

factors distinguish one form of dementia from another. Consequently, when a person is presented with a diagnosis of Alzheimer's disease, often one of the first questions posed by the patient or family is: "What exactly is Alzheimer's disease, and how is it different from dementia?" It is useful to review the definition of dementia, because AD is a form of dementia.

According to Mesulam

M. Marsel-Mesulam, an esteemed behavioral neurologist from Northwestern University, has defined dementia as a "progressive decline in intellect and/or comportment, which causes a gradual restriction of customary daily living activities unrelated to changes of alertness, mobility, or sensorium." At first, this explanation may seem overwhelming, but it becomes more manageable when each part is considered separately. Additionally, it is important to keep in mind that this is a definition of a *clinical syndrome*. This means that, initially, the most relevant information comes from the patient's medical, occupational, and social history, as opposed to the lab tests or radiologic procedures that may be necessary later.

The first part of Mesulam's definition states that dementia is a "progressive decline in intellect...." *Progressive* refers to the time course of the illness. With regard to dementia, changes are generally noticed over months to years, as opposed to hours or days. The word *progressive* is important, because a person with AD, for example, tends to gradually but steadily decline. On the other hand, a relatively sudden intellectual decline in a previously normal person is not likely the result of dementia, but rather of some other medical condition, such as a stroke or drug intoxication.

The next word in Mesulam's definition is *decline*. This word distinguishes dementia from mental retardation, which occurs at or near birth. Dementia is an acquired condition whereby a person has attained a certain level of intellectual achievement, which then changes for the worse. That does not mean that mentally retarded people are immune to dementia. In fact, the observation that people with Down's syndrome may experience a decline in cognitive ability as they live into their 30s and 40s (the upper end of their life expectancy) is an important clue to understanding the development of AD. Sometimes it can be difficult to distinguish if a person with baseline low intelligence and/or limited education has a superimposed dementia. In these situations, careful documentation of the person's previous achievements is critical to decide whether a decline in their abilities has, in fact, occurred.

The last word in this part of the definition is *intellect*. Intellectual abilities include a collection of cognitive functions that may be affected separately in dementia. *Cognitive function* refers to memory, language, spatial reasoning, and executive function, among others. Within each cognitive domain there are various subdomains that can also be differentially affected by the disease. For example, memory is often divided into sensory, short-term, and long-term. *Executive function* refers to the ability to plan ahead, understand future consequences, and make appropriate decisions. Clinicians use bedside tests of mental status to get a rough idea of a person's abilities in these different areas. A more in depth examination may be requested, however, over the course of the illness.

Mesulam not only includes intellect, but *comportment* as something that can be affected either alone or in addition to the aforementioned intellectual domains. In general, *comportment* refers to a person's behavior during social interactions. Appropriate responses in social situations require normal functioning of the frontal lobes of the brain. One of the more common non-Alzheimer's dementias that affects social reasoning abilities is called *frontotemporal dementia*. The first symptoms of Pick's disease, one type of frontotemporal dementia, are specific problems related to social behaviors, while leaving other intellectual abilities initially unaffected.

These changes or a decline in social and/or intellectual properties in turn "cause a gradual restriction of customary daily living activities...." Although it is not easy to precisely define the activities of daily living,

> Changes or a decline in social and/or intellectual properties cause a gradual restriction of customary daily living activities.

this important component is necessary for the diagnosis of dementia. It prevents people from being labeled *demented* just because they have difficulties solving complex mental problems, but report no problems in conducting their day-to-day activities. Unfortunately, deciding exactly how much deterioration in a person's ability to balance a checkbook, drive a car, or plan a shopping trip, for example, is necessary for the diagnosis of dementia has proved complicated. Certainly, at some point it becomes painfully obvious that a person is impaired in these abilities, but the boundary between normal and impaired is a fuzzy one.

The degree of deterioration is not the only difficult decision involved in diagnosis; the use of the term *customary* may differ significantly from one person to the next. For instance, an individual regularly participating in more demanding activities, such as their job, may notice more subtle changes when they occur. Another individual may have to experience rather substantial declines in ability before recognizing their importance. Regardless, it is clear that the dementing process must have started before it reached the point where it began to affect daily activities. It may go undiagnosed or even unnoticed, however, until daily living skills are impacted.

Lastly, Mesulam notes that the restriction in daily living activity is "unrelated to changes of alertness, mobility, or sensorium." These three exclusions are crucial for ruling out other possible diagnoses. The first exclusion, and perhaps the most important, regards *alertness*. Alertness provides the key distinction between dementia and delirium. *Delirium* is an acute confused state characterized by fluctuating levels of alertness, hallucinations, and alterations in sleep-wake cycles, among other symptoms. It is most commonly seen in the hospital setting, and elderly patients are at high risk for developing delirium. Many causes may account for a delirious state, including the effects of medication, infections, and alterations of body chemistries, such as sodium and calcium blood levels. Delirium is reversible with the correction of underlying problems, as opposed to dementia, which, except in relatively rare circumstances, cannot be reversed. Unfortunately, patients with dementia are especially susceptible to delirium, often complicating treatment.

The second and third exclusions refer to mobility and sensorium—meaning "of the senses." A person who suffers from a medical condition that limits mobility (for example, arthritis) may have some trouble performing daily tasks. Likewise, poor vision may also limit activities such as driving or balancing a checkbook. These limitations should not be confused with the problems of conducting customary daily living activities resulting from dementia. Unfortunately, the process of sorting out responsibility can be complicated by multiple potential causes. For example, someone who has arthritis and vision loss may also suffer some cognitive impairment that limit activities.

Alzheimer's Disease Definition According to the *Diagnostic and Statistical Manual*

The *Diagnostic and Statistical Manual, 4th Edition* (DSM-IV), published by the American Psychiatric Association, has officially recommended a set of criteria for Alzheimer's disease that has been widely endorsed. These criteria pose a major problem for the clinician, however, because it requires that a person have *both* memory and at least one additional cognitive disturbance in order to be diagnosed with AD. This is more restrictive than Mesulam's definition, which simply requires a decline in intellect, but does not specify any further characterization of the deficits. The difficulty in using the DSM-IV's criteria centers on a group of patients who have a clear gradual decline in memory, sufficient to cause disability, but no other demonstrable cognitive disturbances. This condition has been called *isolated amnestic syndrome*. However, upon postmortem examination, many of these patients have been proved to have AD, although, on occasion, other diseases such as small strokes may be present.

The DSM-IV's more restrictive criteria may also affect patients in the early stages of AD. In some cases, the diagnosis of AD is not given because only memory deficits are present; but with time, other symptoms develop that warrant an AD diagnosis. This has the unfortunate side effect of postponing treatment in a disease where increasing evidence suggests that early intervention is important. On a more positive note, by investigating purely amnestic syndromes as possible precursors to AD, researchers may learn about the early phases of the illness and perhaps improve treatment during this period.

According to the NINCDS

These problems are largely avoided in the NINCDS-ADRDA (National Institute of Neurologic and Communicable Diseases-Alzheimer's Disease and Related Disorders Association) diagnostic criteria for AD, which distinguish between *probable* and *possible* AD. (There is no *definite* AD in their classification apart from autopsy or biopsy-confirmed AD.) Patients with deficits in just one cognitive area, such as memory, would be classified as possible AD; whereas those with deficits in two or more areas qualify for probable AD. Incidentally, unlike Mesulam and the DSM-IV definitions, impaired activities of daily living are considered supportive, not required, features of an AD diagnosis. In common with the other proposed diagnostic criteria, progressive worsening and absence of disturbance of consciousness are required.

ALZHEIMER'S IS THE MOST COMMON TYPE OF DEMENTIA

There are many possible causes of dementia besides AD, including *Lewy body dementia*, frontotemporal dementia, and *vascular dementia*, as well as various neurologic and medical conditions, such as brain tumors or certain vitamin deficiencies that may cause dementia (see Chapter 6). However, studies concur that AD is by far the most common type of dementia, accounting for approximately 60 percent of cases. Vascular dementia (from stroke) is the second most common, comprising about 25 percent, and the remaining 15 percent of the dementia population is composed of patients with various other diseases. AD is definitively distinguished from other types of dementia by the findings in the brain on autopsy (see Chapter 7), but there are many clues that allow a physician to distinguish AD from other diseases while the patient is alive.

Chapter 2

Normal Aging versus Alzheimer's

Chapter Question:
His memory is slipping—is he just getting old
or is it Alzheimer's?

Distinguishing the deterioration of cognitive function that may occur with normal aging from the early signs of Alzheimer's disease is challenging, but there are clues that can help us. Chapter 2 discusses the difference between healthy aging, normal aging, and pathologic aging, and reviews the term *mild cognitive impairment* and its relationship to AD.

NORMAL AGING AND COGNITION

YOU ANSWER HER QUESTION and 5 minutes later she asks the same question again. It took him half an hour to locate his car in the mall parking lot. The name of an old acquaintance is on the tip of her tongue, but she cannot quite remember what it is. We all experience these little lapses in memory from time to time. In most cases, they represent a trivial, temporary failure in our recall abilities. But if memory lapses and cognitive oversights happen on a regular basis in an older person, they may be early warning signs of AD.

Historically, aging has been considered synonymous with cognitive decline, especially memory loss. However, we now know that significant deterioration of cognition is not inevitable. There are many anecdotal examples of individuals living up to a century or more with little or no cognitive changes. Researchers have also been able to demonstrate that people age differently, some experiencing few changes in their abilities, while others suffer more considerable losses, and perhaps even develop AD.

One outcome of these studies has been the development of a three-category classification of aging with respect to cognitive function: healthy aging, normal aging, and pathologic aging. In general, *healthy aging* refers to people who have minimal or no medical problems, take few or no prescription medications, and remain active socially, physically, and intellectually. *Normal aging* identifies the more common course among aging persons, including those who have been diagnosed with a variety of chronic illnesses, such as diabetes, hypertension, arthritis, or coronary artery disease. They may take several prescription medications, and may see some change in the intensity and frequency of the leisure and social activities they previously enjoyed. Last, *pathologic aging* describes those individuals who suffer greater changes in their cognitive abilities. They may have trouble performing day-to-day activities, and will develop a disease process such as AD or some other dementia.

Categorizing an older person as healthy or normal can be problematic. No one can anticipate the future, and people who may be deemed normal at one point in time may eventually develop a pathologic illness later in life. For example, in 2000, the Oregon Brain Aging Study published its findings from 95 individuals over the age of 84 years. At the beginning of the investigation, all of the participants were deemed "healthy elder" because they suffered from no medical or psychological illnesses. After 13 years, 25 percent had developed AD; 25 percent had decreased but not pathologic test scores; and a full 50 percent showed no change in test results. Although these results are encouraging in their documentation that cognitive decline is not an inevitable consequence of aging, it also reminds us that the classification of "healthy elder" is not necessarily stable, and studies of aging should never assume that these classifications will not change.

Once a person is considered a "normal elder," he is included in a higher-risk group for developing pathologic processes. For instance, people with cardiovascular disease have a greater chance of developing AD, whcreas diabetics may develop the memory loss associated with shrink-age of the *hippocampus*. The hippocampus is an area of the brain that is important in memory formation, as we'll explore in more detail in the next chapter.

COGNITION AND AGING

Before turning to a discussion of pathologic aging, it is important to con-sider in more detail the question of what occurs to cognition in the course of normal aging. This is not an easy question to answer. Some of the results of past studies on this topic have to be heavily discounted or thrown out altogether, because the groups of elderly people used in these studies often inadvertently included people with undiagnosed mild or even moderate AD. These were patients whose poorer scores decreased the average of the normal elderly. Even today, it is still diffi-cult, if not impossible, to be certain that a group of "normal" elderly patients does not include people with undetected early AD. For exam-ple, a study published in *Neurology* showed that people with low scores on a test of visual memory were more likely to be diagnosed with AD *10 years later*! These people probably would have been classified as normal had they been asked to serve in a study of normal aging. Yet, in all like-lihood, their brains were already harboring AD lesions that were respon-sible for their relatively low scores on the visual memory test, and this could therefore have affected their performance on other tests as well. This problem of defining "normal" becomes increasingly vexing as researchers start looking at people in their 70s and up, because the prevalence of AD increases relentlessly with advancing age. As a result, researchers are more and more likely to include some of the early symp-tomatic group in what they thought were healthy controls.

Another example that shows how thinking has evolved in this area was pointed out in a study that appeared in the December 2003 issue of *Neurology*. This study examined *spatial disorientation* (the tendency to become lost) in AD. Four groups were studied: young normals, middle-aged normals, older nondemented people (average age 73), and mild AD patients. The subjects were led around a particular path in a large hospital lobby. Then they had to retrace the path and answer various questions about it, such as whether they turned right or left at a certain point, what landmarks were visible along the path, and so on. Their performance of these tasks was compared to results on a battery of neuropsychological tests. It was found, unsurprisingly, that young and middle-aged people did best; AD patients did worst; and the older group was in between. Formerly, the conclusion would have been that a tendency to get lost was a normal part of aging, but the study went further. The older group was subdivided into those who performed normally on the spatial task and those who did not. Although there was no difference in these subgroups in their performance of the other cognitive tests, the types of errors made in the spatial performance task by the impaired older group was the same as those made by the AD patients; for example, misidentifying a picture as being taken along the route, when, in fact, it was taken somewhere else. The conclusion drawn by the researchers was not that problems with spatial orientation are a natural part of aging, but rather that the subgroup of older people with problems in this area might have a spatial variant of mild cognitive impairment, which, as we will see shortly, is often a prelude to AD.

Be that as it may, most researchers in this area agree that some areas of cognition do show deterioration as a normal result of aging. The brain, like all our other organ systems, was not designed for immortality! Individuals going through the normal aging process tend to experience reduced processing speed, slower reaction times, and some trouble with short-term memory, such as the ability to repeat a phone number after a few minutes have passed. Several studies suggest caution, however, in the interpretation of some previous cognitive aging investigations. Even with the seemingly obvious reduction in processing speed that occurs with aging, some qualifications may be in order. For example, Pichora-Fuller measured the spoken language comprehension of young adults, but altered the speech to simulate how an elderly person with some hearing loss might perceive speech. They reported a slowing of the comprehension abilities in the young adults that was almost the same as in much older individuals. They concluded that, in some cases, the cognitive slowing seen in elderly patients may be accounted for by deficits in hearing or vision. The field of defining more precisely what occurs to cognition during the normal aging process remains a very active area of investigation.

MILD COGNITIVE IMPAIRMENT

At a given point in time, the distinction between healthy and normal aging may be relatively straightforward. Distinguishing normal from pathologic can be difficult, however, especially when the person experiences only mild symptoms as a result of the early stage of an illness. The

> The term *mild cognitive impairment* (MCI) is used when initial symptoms become noticeable, but the consequences do not interfere with the ability to function.

term *mild cognitive impairment* (MCI) is used when these initial symptoms become noticeable, but the consequences do not interfere with the ability to function. The illness progresses from a phase in which there are no symptoms to MCI, and then to the full-blown illness in which symptoms include the inability to perform certain tasks. Researchers are striving to understand this process in AD in hopes of identifying preventive strategies, early warning signs, and effective treatments

To help expose this degenerative process, it is important for doctors and scientists to be able to correctly identify individuals experiencing MCI. Closely related concepts in the literature are *age-associated memory impairment* (AAMI) and *cognitively impaired not demented* (CIND). For practical purposes, despite fine distinctions in definitions, people in these categories appear to be largely the same as those diagnosed as MCI. In 1999, Ron Petersen published five criteria of MCI, which up until recently had become the largely accepted definition of mild cognitive impairment (see Table 2-1). Items four and five are the most accepted criteria, whereas the first three criteria have generated some resistance.

Table 2-1: Petersen Criteria for Mild Cognitive Impairment (MCI)

1. Subjective memory complaint by patient or informant
2. Objective memory impairment for age and education
3. Largely intact general cognitive function
4. Essentially preserved activites of daily living
5. Not demented

Note: Adopted from Petersen, R. (1999). Mild cognitive impairment. *Archives of Neurology*, 56, 303-308.

Criterion 1, that a subjective memory complaint must be present, is perhaps the most controversial. In practice, a memory complaint by the patient is often a better predictor of depression than an actual memory deficit. Many pathologic patients are unaware of their memory loss. Family members or close friends may notice the changes and, hopefully, report them to the physician. At least two studies, one led by Tabert and one led by Carr, have shown that a mismatch in perception of memory loss between the patient and family members is, in itself, a predictor of progression to AD. The take-home message from this is: If you notice a clear problem in your loved one, but she denies it, the odds are very high *that you are right and she has a problem*!

Unfortunately, even family members can be oblivious to memory decline. In 1997, Ross and colleagues published a study reporting that among mild dementia patients, 52 percent of participating families were unaware of the patient's memory problem.

Criterion 2, that an objective memory impairment must be present, has posed more of a practical than theoretical problem. An objective memory score must be obtained from a standardized memory test, such as the Wechsler Memory Test. A person performing 1.5 standard deviations below the mean might be considered impaired. For example, if the mean on a test is 100 and the standard deviation is 10, a person scoring an 80 might be considered impaired because he achieved less than 85, which is 1.5 standard deviations from the mean. Most available objective memory measures can take up to an hour to administer, and there is no agreement on which memory test is best for judging MCI. Until these practical problems are solved, it may difficult for a physician to make an informed decision about criterion 2.

Lastly, criterion 3, that the patient must have largely intact general cognitive function, presents an exclusion problem that has since been addressed with a more specific classification system. Petersen's criterion 3 has caused his definition of MCI to be classified instead as a subtype of MCI, termed *amnestic MCI*, because it requires memory impairment to be the one and only cognitive area affected for diagnosis. The term *non-amnestic MCI* is used to refer to patients who have deficits in other cognitive areas but no impairment of memory. Finally, patients who meet all four other criteria and have both memory and other cognitive deficits are classified as having *multiple cognitive deficit MCI*. Whether there are differences in outcome for these proposed subtypes of MCI is not yet clear. There is one study, however, reporting that amnestic MCI leads to AD, whereas selective impairment in executive function may be an early sign of vascular dementia.

Prevalence and Outcome in MCI

The prevalence estimates of MCI depend upon how it is defined and what population is studied. The Cardiovascular Health Study, which included amnestic and multiple cognitive deficit MCI, reported a 29 percent prevalence rate in those over 85 years old. A second study, published by Busse, used various definitions of MCI, and found that the prevalence rates varied from 3 to 20 percent, depending upon the definition used. In both studies, if the controversial criterion 1 (subjective memory impairment) was eliminated, the prevalence rates were substantially higher, but the rate of pathologic progression was the same.

Pathologic progression for MCI patients, although not inevitable, is more likely. A large Canadian study by Tuokko reported that 47 percent of about 800 MCI patients developed AD over 5 years, compared with only 15 percent of a similar-sized, no cognitive impairment group. Numerous other studies have found that approximately 10 to 20 percent of MCI patients convert to pathologic (AD) each year. These high AD rates among MCI patients have led some to suggest a strong relationship between MCI and AD. In fact, John Morris and colleagues published an article in 2001 claiming that MCI represents early-stage AD. Their team presented autopsy reports of MCI patients showing the plaques and tangles that are diagnostic of AD (reviewed in Chapter 7). Although this evidence strongly suggests an association, it is by no means a certainty. As many as half of all MCI patients will not progress to AD, and some (up to one-fourth) even go on to show improvement.

This brings up a really interesting question. What if Dr. Morris is right, and basically all MCI patients have AD brain pathology? Is there something different biologically about those who progress versus those who do not? Typically, AD patients get inexorably worse over time. Could the nonprogressive or improving patients have some process going on that has somehow stopped the disease in its tracks? If so, what is it? Can it be harnessed and used therapeutically, or were these patients really normal all along, and just misclassified as MCI initially? Clearly this subgroup of MCI patients deserves careful study.

Based on these prevalence and outcome rates, the American Academy of Neurology (AAN) recommends that patients diagnosed with MCI be monitored for cognitive and functional decline. Evaluations should be conducted every 6 to 12 months, unless specific concerns justify more frequent visits. Physicians who adhere to this schedule greatly increase their chances of recognizing changes in mental status and other signs of disease progression that may warrant treatment.

SCREENING FOR DEMENTIA

If you think about it, some of the issues we have raised in these past few pages are of great concern. A significant proportion of older people have MCI, and yet they (and often their families) are not aware of it. These people are at high risk of progressing to full-blown dementia. The situation with MCI and early dementia may be analogous to having a precancerous lesion, or even having developed cancer, yet having it go undiagnosed and untreated. However, doctors do not routinely screen people for dementia or cognitive impairment. If the patient seems superficially normal, which is very often true for MCI, and even early AD patients, most doctors will not request any testing. Many studies have shown that primary care doctors routinely miss the diagnosis of mild AD, much less MCI. The problem is further exacerbated by the fact that some insurance companies do not cover cognitive testing because the problems discovered are classified as a "nervous or mental disorder," which many policies exclude from reimbursement. This is as out-of-date as the term *nervous disorder*, which does not refer to anxiety, but rather is a nineteenth century term for a psychiatric disease.

One might argue, with some justification, that the identification of patients with MCI is not terribly important, because there is no known effective treatment at this time. Yet, this situation may not hold for long because many trials are being conducted, the goal of which is to delay the progression of MCI to AD (some of these trials are discussed in more detail in Chapter 16). If a treatment for MCI is identified, even if it is only partially effective, the public health benefit is potentially huge, because such a high percentage of the older population is affected.

TO SCREEN OR NOT TO SCREEN, THAT IS THE QUESTION

So, should older people be routinely screened for dementia in the same way that they are screened for hypertension? Although not everybody agrees, there are some strong arguments in favor of screening. Let us

> Should older people be routinely screened for dementia in the same way that they are screened for hypertension?

consider first what makes a disease worth screening for. Table 2-2 lists standard criteria a disease should meet in order to merit screening.

The first criterion is that the disease should be reasonably common in the population. Obviously, if the disease affects only one person in a million, it probably is not going to be cost effective to put 999,999 people through some sort of test to pick up that one case, still no one will argue with the proposition that dementia and MCI are common in the older population.

Table 2-2: Criteria for a Disease to Merit Screening

- Common in the population
- Symptoms not obvious
- Treatment is available
- Early treatment is more beneficial than later treatment
- Effective, safe, and inexpensive screening tool available
- Consequences of misdiagnosing normal people should not outweigh the benefits of correctly diagnosing the truly affected

The second criterion is that symptoms of the disease should not be obvious to the patient. There is no point in making everybody go through a strip search to look for signs of psoriasis, for example, because people are all too aware of the symptoms themselves. As we have discussed in detail, however, the symptoms of early dementia are commonly missed by the patient or the family. The diagnosis of early dementia is also routinely missed by physicians, because patients may appear normal even though they would perform poorly on cognitive testing.

The third criterion is that treatment must be available. Although this used to be the case for AD, fortunately it is no longer true. There is no major harm in delaying the diagnosis of a disease if the outcome is the same whether you treat it sooner versus later. There is mounting evidence that it is more beneficial to treat AD earlier rather than later (see Chapter 9).

A screening tool must be available that is inexpensive, safe and easy to use, and effective in finding people who need further analysis. Although doctors may ask their patients if their blood pressure is okay, they never take the patient's word for it. Blood pressure is always measured during office visits. Analogous measuring tools for dementia exist, which we'll discuss in more detail in Chapter 4.

Finally, the consequences of misdiagnosing normal people should not outweigh the benefits of correctly diagnosing the truly afflicted. If, for example, the treatment for dementia involved some sort of expensive and highly toxic chemotherapy, it would be a serious mistake to put a normal person through that unnecessarily. Fortunately, the available treatments for dementia are not overly expensive and have only minor side effects, which are readily reversible by stopping treatment. Treating a person who does not need it, although regrettable, will not cause any serious long-term effects.

There is also the problem of misdiagnosed people suffering emotional reactions from believing they have AD, when, in fact, they do *not* have AD. On the other hand, most of the diagnostic "mistakes" are likely to be made in distinguishing normal from MCI, and MCI from AD, rather than normal from AD. Given that many patients with MCI progress to AD, misclassifying them as AD at the outset may actually benefit them, in that follow-up will be provided. Plus, although we do not know this yet for sure, treating MCI patients with AD drugs may actually be beneficial. A little more problematic would be diagnosing a normal patient as MCI. But even here, all that would likely happen is simply that the patient will be asked to revisit the physician, and subsequent testing would catch the error. It therefore seems reasonable to conclude that the possible harm caused by misdiagnosing some normal people as MCI, or MCI as demented, would be outweighed by the significant benefits experienced by patients who are diagnosed early and treated appropriately.

The U.S. Preventive Services Task Force published a review of the literature on screening for dementia in 2003, concluding that although the concept was a good one, further research was needed before an official policy was put in place. The American Academy of Neurology, when it examined the screening question a few years ago, similarly concluded that not enough evidence existed to mandate it. However, although clearly more research is needed, many doctors may find the current evidence sufficient for them to begin screening elderly patients using one or more of the specific tests outlined in Chapter 4.

We have now finished discussing in some detail the fuzzy boundary between normal aging and mild cognitive impairment, and it is time to move on to the next fuzzy boundary: the boundary between MCI and AD.

WARNING SIGNS OF ALZHEIMER'S DISEASE

As reviewed in Chapter 1, the transition to AD is defined by the development of problems performing the activities of daily living. Deciding that periodic memory problems have progressed from MCI to AD requires the judgment of a trained physician. There are warning signs, however, that family and friends should notice and report to the doctor. The most important of these is that "things are getting worse." Often in AD, family members and/or the patient will recognize that memory or thinking abilities are gradually getting worse over a period of months,

> There are warning signs that family and friends should notice and report to the doctor.

with changes becoming especially obvious from year to year. But it is not uncommon for a patient to already be in the early phase of AD by the time a family member first feels memory lapses are an actual problem. Often, some specific shocking incident of forgetfulness brings the matter forcibly to attention. Similarly, when a definite change for the worse is noted, the patient may have crossed the boundary into AD. As a rule of thumb, it is highly probable that when a family member first notes memory lapses, the patient is already in the MCI stage, and by the time a definite change for the worse is noted, the patient has already crossed the boundary into AD.

The Alzheimer's Foundation of America and the Alzheimer's Association have distributed similar lists of the symptoms of early stage AD. Table 2-3 is a combination of these warning signs.

Changes in memory are perhaps the most important and the most frequently noticed. The loved one asks a question and it is answered, but then she asks the same question several minutes later. Sometimes, he may forget the details of a conversation, or even that the conversation took place. A common example is getting lost while driving in a familiar area. This is a profound indication that something may be wrong, and the person may need to be evaluated for the ability to drive safely.

Two other early warning signs are loss of initiative and lack of sound judgment. The doctor should be told if a family member becomes apathetic and less involved in previously enjoyed social activities. Apathy

Table 2-3: Early Warning Signs of AD

1. Forgetting things more often
   Example: names, telephone numbers, recent events, misplacing items
2. Becoming confused about time and place
   Example: getting lost trying to find own home
3. Having problems with routine task
   Example: buttoning a shirt, boiling an egg
4. Experiencing erratic changes in mood or behavior
   Example: easily angered or depressed
5. Having trouble communicating
   Example forgetting common words, using the wrong words
6. Experiencing changes in personality
   Example: feeling afraid or suspicious
7. Loss of initiative
8. Problems with abstract thinking
9. Lack of sound judgment
   Example: wearing inappropriate clothes for the season

Note: Adapted from *Signs and Symptoms* distributed by the Alzheimer's Association and the Alzheimer's Foundation of America.

can occur in depression, but is also a sign of pathologic aging. Likewise, errors in judgment should be investigated by a physician. Unfortunately, unless the person is regularly confronted with major decisions or engaged in fairly demanding activities, such as running their own business, this sign may go unnoticed for quite some time. Many a nice, slightly demented widow has been fleeced of her life savings by a smooth-talking con artist who has convinced her of a "once-in-a-lifetime" investment opportunity.

Lastly, the signs that often occur in mild to moderate stages of AD are difficulties with routine tasks, changes in behavior, mood, or personality, and problems with language. As with other signs of AD, these could be explained by a variety of other causes. If a person is experiencing multiple symptoms, and the problems are getting worse over time, then it is more likely that he will be diagnosed as having AD.

One tool that the doctor may ask a caregiver or family member to complete is the Functional Activities Questionnaire (FAQ). This is a short form by which the patient is rated by the observer on a variety of daily tasks using a 0–3 scale. The tasks include handling finances, shopping, cooking, keeping track of current events, and remembering appointments. The FAQ can be a powerful tool for the physician to document the transition from MCI to AD, where demonstration of impairment in the performance of daily activities is necessary, and to evaluate the patient's response to treatment.

Chapter 3

How Memory Works

Chapter Question:
Why can she remember her high school graduation,
but not her current daily appointments?

Memory can be divided into sensory, short-term, and long-term memory. Long-term memory is further divided into conscious (declarative) and unconscious (nondeclarative) memory. Alzheimer's disease pathology tends to begin in the hippocampus and *entorhinal cortex*. Because short-term memory requires these brain areas, problems with it are usually among the first and most prominent of AD symptoms.

> Memory can be divided into sensory, short-term, and long-term memory.

IINTRODUCTION TO PATIENT H.M.

IT HAS BEEN SAID that memory is the only known process that can reverse "time's arrow," allowing us to perform mental time travel into our past. The modern era of memory research began in 1953, with the story of H.M., who was in his early twenties and suffering from severe seizures when Dr. William Scoville decided to try a new surgical procedure in an attempt to stop them. He removed part of each temporal lobe, including most of the hippocampus. The procedure was a success in that H.M.'s seizures became rare events, and he was able to cut down on his anticonvulsant medications. Shortly after recovering from the operation, however, it was noted that he was unable to form new memories.

23

H.M. has normal general intelligence and preserved social skills, but if you shake hands with him, walk out of the room, and come back a few moments later, he will not recognize you. He does not remember any life events since his operation. He cannot explain the meanings of words that have become common in the last 60 years, such as "granola" or "Jacuzzi." He has no trouble performing new tasks that require motor skills, such as tracing an object reflected by a mirror, although each time he claims he has never done the task before. The numerous studies of H.M., and many other patients suffering similar lesions or damage, have contributed to a greater understanding of memory systems and how they are formed and maintained.

THREE-STAGE MEMORY MODEL

Memory is typically classified by the time between an event and its recall. The most accepted memory structure, the three-stage model, includes sensory memory (recall in milliseconds to seconds); short-term and working memory (recall in seconds to minutes); and long-term memory (recall in hours to years). Furthermore, memory can be conscious, also known as declarative memory, or unconscious, nondeclarative memory. Figure 3-1 illustrates the three-stage model. Figure 3-2 reviews conscious and unconscious memory types.

Sensory Memory

Imagine that you are at a football game, and a friend has been telling you about his new job. You have not really been listening because you are watching the game. Your friend says suddenly, "Did you hear what I just said?" You immediately review in your head what he was just say-

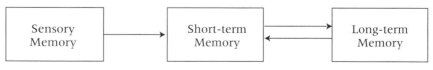

FIGURE 3-1

Three-stage memory model. Note: Adapted from figures by Alan Baddeley.

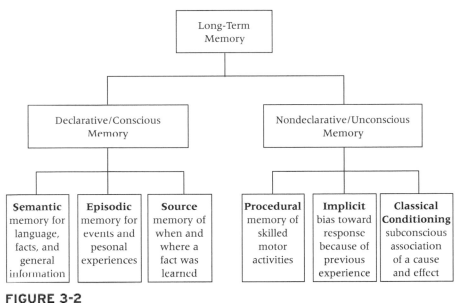

FIGURE 3-2

Long-term memory.

ing, even though you were not paying attention, and you are able to repeat it back to him. Had he asked you a few minutes after he said it, however, you would not have been able to recall it.

Sensory memory only lasts a very short time. It is forgotten almost immediately, unless there is some reason to pay attention to it. Consequently, the storage and retrieval of sensory experiences is highly dependent upon expectation, attention, and general arousal state. For

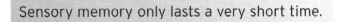
Sensory memory only lasts a very short time.

example, in an experiment by Daniel Simons and Christopher Chabris, normal young adults watched a video clip of people playing basketball, and were told to count the number of passes. A woman in a gorilla suit strolled across the scene in plain view about half-way through the clip. When asked if they had seen anything unusual during the presentation, almost everyone said no. When asked specifically if they recalled seeing a woman in a gorilla suit, most of them still did not recall the event.

Their attention was focused on the basketball game, and since they had not been told to watch for anything unusual, they did not pay attention to (or store in short-term memory) the woman in the gorilla suit.

Short-Term Memory

Experiences are stored and retrieved from short-term, working memory, under the attention of the individual. Short-term memory lasts longer than sensory memory. It has a limited capacity of 7±2 (read seven

> Short-term memory lasts longer than sensory memory.

plus or minus two) chunks, however. A chunk can be one item, such as the number of things needed at the store, or several items, such as the area code of a telephone number. The older memories get "pushed out" when this limited capacity is exceeded.

People use short-term memory when actively trying to solve a problem, or when trying to store items in long-term memory. In problem solving, one may need the *visuospatial sketch pad*, an imagery tool of working memory. For example, if asked whether a cat's tail is longer than 18 inches, one might imagine a cat's tail with a yardstick next to it and realize that generally cat's tails are shorter than 18 inches. On the other hand, if it is necessary to remember a phone number while waiting to use the telephone, one might utilize the *phonological* or *rehearsal loop*. People use this working memory tool when they repeat something over and over again to themselves in order to remember it.

Working memory can be crudely tested during a regular office visit. The patient may be asked to recall a series of numbers in reversed order, spell a word backwards, or alphabetize a short list of words without writing them down. The most difficult tests for AD patients are tests of short-term memory involving a delay of a few minutes between the initial *encoding*—when, for example, three words that they are told to remember are repeated—and subsequent *recall*, often after some distracting task is done to prevent them from using strategies such as the phonological loop to keep the items in mind.

Long-Term Memory

Items that are attended to and deemed important may get stored in long-term memory. Once an item or experience is stored in long-term memory, it may stay there forever. There is no limit to how many memories can be stored, and recall may be from hours to decades after the event. The process of recalling stored memories is not always easy, and

> **Long-term memories may last forever.**

search strategies and memory structures differ from person to person. For example, an individual may not have thought about his grandmother's old house for 20 years, but then one day he meets a person wearing the perfume she wore when he was a child. Detailed memories of the house and his grandmother may suddenly be remembered. In this example, the man may have never been able to remember the smell of his grandmother's perfume, or exactly where her wedding picture hung in the house, but the smell of this new woman's perfume triggered the memory paths that allowed him to remember a great number of details. Long-term memories vary widely in the way they are learned or experienced, and in the ways they can be retrieved. Figure 3-2 is an illustration of how experts classify long-term memory based on these storage and retrieval processes.

Conscious or Declarative Memory

Declarative memory refers to memories that are consciously learned or stored and actively retrieved. Episodic memory and semantic memory are the two main types of declarative memory, but source memory also falls into the declarative category. *Episodic memory* refers to memories of particular events in our lives; for example, a person's high school graduation, the time she scored the winning goal, or his first kiss. *Semantic memory*, on the other hand, refers to specific facts that we have acquired about the world over the years; for example, that George Washington was the first president, whales live in the ocean, or that forks and knives are used at the dinner table. In most cases, it is impossible to remember where or when these facts were first learned. Remembering the context of when something was learned is called *source memory*; for example, where you were when you first learned that the World Trade Center was hit on September 11, 2001.

Unconscious or Nondeclarative Memory

The complement to conscious memory is *unconscious or nondeclarative memory*. Unconscious memories do not always require attention for learning or storage, and their retrieval is effortless. These memory processes include procedural memory, implicit memory, and classical conditioning, which is a form of learning. Procedural memory refers to learned motor skills, such as how to ride a bike or drive a car. When first learning these skills, a person may be aware of some of the things he is doing, but in time the motions become automatic.

Implicit memory also does not require especially attentive storage processes, but it generally involves non–motor learning. For example, a person is asked to read a list of words (such as "chair, mouse, bandit, frog") with no instructions to remember them. Later, if they are asked to recall the words on the list, they will probably not remember them. If they are asked to complete the word stem "mo" to make a word, however, they are more likely to respond with "mouse," which was on the word list, instead of "more," "most," or any other words that start with "mo." Even though they did not remember the word "mouse" from the list well enough to recall it, there was a least a trace of the word in memory that was strong enough to bias their word stem completion.

The third type of unconscious memory is a result of *classical conditioning*, which occurs when an association between two items or experiences becomes learned without the conscious effort of the learner. The best example of classical conditioning comes from the Russian psychologist who discovered it, Ivan Pavlov, who studied the digestive system of dogs. Before each feeding, he rang a bell to signal that the meat was coming. Over time, he noticed that the dogs would begin salivating when the bell was rung, well before the meat was presented. Unwittingly, he had "conditioned" the dogs to salivate to a sound by associating it with meat. Using another example from the digestive system, humans may experience this type of learning if they get sick shortly after eating a certain food. The next time they encounter that particular food, they may get a little queasy and not want to eat it.

MEMORY FORMATION

The complete explanation of memory formation is complex. Consequently, this discussion will focus on a memory structure important in Alzheimer's disease, the *hippocampus*. Figure 3-3 is a side view of the brain, showing the cortex (lighter part) surrounding the primitive parts of the brain (darker), many of which are important for memory formation. The hippocampus appears towards the bottom of the drawing.

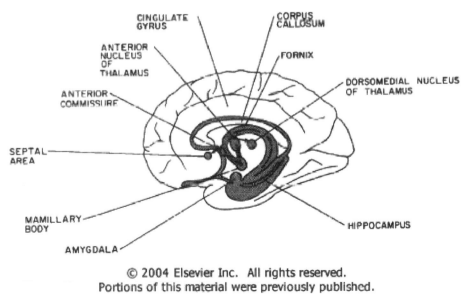

FIGURE 3-3

Subcortical structures involved in memory.

and is considered below the cortex, or *subcortical*. These subcortical structures form communication networks with one another, as well as with parts of the *cortex* (lobes of the brain). You will note the *amygdala*, another *subcortical nucleus*, in close proximity to the hippocampus. The amygdala is important in emotional reactions. Ask yourself, what events in your life do you tend to remember? You will probably find that most of them caused some sort of emotional reaction in you at the time, be it good or bad. The amygdala's connections with the hippocampus help to cement in memory events that are emotionally important. The amygdala activates the hippocampus and instructs it to turn your present experience into a memory. The *dorsomedial nucleus* of the *thalamus* is another important structure for memory. Alcoholics who have *Korsakoff's psychosis*—a disease characterized by severe and relatively selective problems with short-term memory—typically have damage to this structure.

Many of these communication systems become activated when the brain is confronted with a series of experiences. As a result of attention, repetition, or the importance of incoming stimuli, certain experiences become stored in memory. During the storage process, the hippocampus puts a "stamp" of sorts on the active communication systems related to the experience. When a memory is retrieved, the whole system becomes reactivated. In practice, this occurs when a person remembers a part of a memory (where the event took place), or searches for a particular part of a memory (the name of cousin Betty's new boyfriend), and then the whole memory is activated along with many of the details (the wedding at cousin Betty's house when you met her new boyfriend). However, when an event is remembered, the actual event cannot be precisely remembered, only reconstructed. This is why we may remember things inaccurately or incompletely. Frequently reactivated circuits are more easily retrieved, but they are also more vulnerable to "rewriting."

The hippocampus is necessary to form new memories, but if it is damaged, old memories may still be retrieved. Conversely, if the hippocampus is intact, but parts of the cerebral cortex are damaged, then new memories can be stored, but old memories may be lost. In AD, the hippocampus begins to suffer damage in the early phases of the illness. Plaques and tangles begin to form here and then spread to other parts of

The hippocampus is necessary to form new memories.

the brain, including the cortex. Consequently, a person with AD has trouble storing new memories, and then begins to have trouble retrieving older memories. The oldest memories are recalled best, while the newer memories begin to fade. The inverse situation is seen in a rare form of dementia called *semantic dementia*. In this disease, early on the hippocampus is relatively intact, but the *temporal cortex*, where semantic information is stored, is damaged. These patients have relatively intact short-term memory, but impaired long-term memory abilities.

NEURAL TRANSMISSION AND MEMORY

As plaques and tangles begin to interfere with the functioning of the hippocampus and other brain areas, the communication system of the brain cells becomes adversely affected. Brain cells, or neurons, communicate via chemical and electrical transmission. The chemicals used by neurons are called *neurotransmitters*; they are necessary for all parts of the brain to function correctly. Neurons release neurotransmitters into the *synaptic clefts*, the small spaces between the neurons. The receiving neuron picks up the neurotransmitter via special *receptors* in the cell membrane. When the "message" is received, the cell is either excited or inhibited. At the basic level, excitation messages may cause the cell to release neurotransmitter to the next cell; whereas inhibition messages may keep that cell from releasing neurotransmitter to the next cell.

Several neurotransmitter systems are affected in AD. Two types of medications that have proved to be promising for AD patients act on the neurotransmitters that are important for learning and memory. The first type of medication affects glutamate transmission; this is represented by the drug memantine (Namenda®). Namenda® works on a glutamate receptor. Glutamate is an excitatory neurotransmitter that is necessary for learning and the formation of long-term memory. The NMDA (N-methyl-D-aspartate) receptor is one type of glutamate receptor. Normal stimulation of the NMDA receptor facilitates learning. Overstimulation of this receptor, however, can cause the cell to become sick or die. Glutamate toxicity resulting from overstimulated NMDA receptors may contribute to AD. Namenda® binds to NMDA receptors and prevents them from becoming overexcited, while still allowing them to function normally in neural communication.

A second type of medication improves acetylcholine transmission; this includes donepezil (Aricept®), arivastigmine (Exelon®), and galantamine (Reminyl®). In the brain, acetylcholine is primarily an excitatory neurotransmitter, and, similar to glutamate, it plays a key role in learning and memory. AD patients generally show large losses in brain areas dense in acetylcholine-producing neurons. These medications increase the amount of acetylcholine available, thus improving functions modulated by this neurotransmitter.

CONCLUSION

There are many different kinds of memory. Alzheimer's disease is a degenerative illness that begins in the brain regions that are important for short-term memory, in particular, and gradually spreads to other areas, affecting the brain's communication systems. AD patients may have trouble forming new memories, but can often remember their oldest memories best because the hippocampus is usually compromised early in the disease. The new drugs that provide some relief of memory impairment to AD patients focus on improving the communications systems that are necessary for learning and memory.

Chapter 4

Diagnosis of Dementia

Chapter Question:
What tests are available for dementia?

The diagnosis of dementia largely relies on clinical interviews
with the patient and family members, because there are no laboratory tests or radiologic studies that can affirm or refute a diagnosis of dementia. There are brief bedside tests of mental status
that may aid in the initial screening of dementia as well as more
extensive neuropsychologic exams, blood tests, and neurodiagnostic tests, such as MRI and *electroencephalogram* (EEG). Chapter
4 reviews some of the different kinds of tests that may be used
in the diagnosis of AD.

BRIEF BEDSIDE TESTS OF MENTAL STATUS

B RIEF TESTS OF MENTAL STATUS can be conducted (3 to 10 minutes) that
provide the neurologist with important information that may lead
to further testing or a fine-tuning of diagnostic considerations. These
tests are not considered diagnostic on their own, but when included as
part of a complete examination, they assist in ruling out or "ruling in"
certain causes. Seven of these exams will be briefly discussed in this
chapter.

The Mini-Mental State Examination

One of the oldest and most widely used bedside tests is the Mini-Mental
State Examination (MMSE), which was developed by Dr. Marshall
Folstein in the mid-1970s. This examination has achieved widespread

acceptance in both the research and clinical communities. The MMSE asks questions covering several areas of cognition, with possible scores ranging from 0 to 30. The first 10 points are earned by answering questions regarding the date and present location. Three points are earned

> One of the oldest and most widely used bedside tests is the Mini-Mental State Examination (MMSE).

for immediate memory (repetition of three items; for example, "apple, table, penny"); 3 points are earned for the recall of these three items. Five points are earned for serially subtracting 7s from 100 (that is, "93-86-79-72-65"), or for correctly spelling a five-letter word backwards. Finally, 9 points are earned for tasks that assess a range of cognitive function, including naming objects, following a three-part instruction, writing a sentence, and copying a figure. In general, scores of 27 or higher are considered normal; scores between 23 and 26 are borderline; and scores 22 or below are abnormal. For AD patients, scores from 20 to 26 correlate to mild AD; scores from 10 to 19, and those less than 10, correspond to moderate and severe AD, respectively.

In AD patients, scores on this exam have been used to predict when certain difficulties might arise over the course of the illness. Figure 4-1 shows the correlation of the loss of ability to perform various activities of daily living with the MMSE score and the number of years since diagnosis. For example, the ability to keep appointments may be lost by one-fourth of those with an initial MMSE score of 25, but after several years, when the MMSE score has dropped to 18, as many as three-fourths of patients have lost this ability. Similarly, the ability to appropriately select clothes is lost by one-fourth of those with MMSE scores of 20 2 years after diagnosis; after 7 years and an MMSE score of 8, three-fourths of patients may have trouble with this task. On average, untreated AD patients lose 2 to 4 points per year on the MMSE.

Unfortunately, the MMSE has two important limitations. First, it is sensitive to education. Highly educated people who are mildly dement-

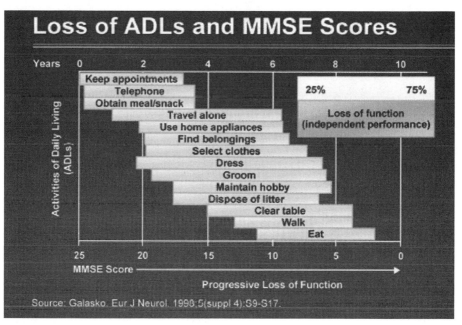

FIGURE 4-1

Correlation of activities of daily living with years since diagnosis and MMSE scores.

ed may still score within the normal range because the questions are too easy for them, but, conversely, poorly educated but cognitively normal people may score in the dementia range because some of the questions are too difficult. Second, some physicians choose not to use this test because it takes too long to administer (5 to 10 minutes).

The Clock Drawing Test

The clock drawing test is a simple, easy to administer exam that is used both as a screening tool and as part of more comprehensive neuropsy-

> The clock drawing test is a simple, easy-to-administer exam, but is not sensitive for detecting early dementia.

chologic testing. The instructions are to "Draw a clock. Put in all the numbers. Set the hands at ten past eleven." This test appears simple but the results can provide a wealth of information related to memory, strategy, vision, and processing of information. Figure 4-2 is a clock drawing from an 85-year-old man who was referred for possible Lou Gehrig's disease (amyotrophic lateral sclerosis). The man and his family denied any problems with memory, but admitted that occasionally he seemed "a little confused."

The patient made several errors. He duplicated the number 12, left out the hands, and wrote "to" in between the 11 and 12 with a little arrow pointing to it (perhaps trying to represent ten to eleven). As a result of this and other testing, as well as conversations with the family, the gentleman was later diagnosed with AD.

Although numerous scoring systems are available for this test, the AD cooperative scoring system has 5 points: 1 for the circle, 1 for all numbers being present in the correct order, 1 for the numbers being in a proper spatial arrangement, 1 for two hands being present, and 1 for the correct time. The drawing in Figure 4-2 would earn a score of 2 (1 for the circle and 1 for the numbers being in a proper spatial arrangement). A normal score is 4 or 5.

The clock drawing test shares a similar criticism with the MMSE: It is not very sensitive to mild impairments. Virtually all normal people will perform well on this test, as will many individuals with mild dementia. When the exam is abnormal, however, it does offer specific clues as to which system is affected.

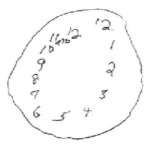

FIGURE 4-2

Example of a clock drawing by an 85-year-old man with AD.

Memory Impairment Screen

Because memory is often one of the earliest and most affected aspects of cognition in AD, it seems reasonable that a screening test focusing on memory would be developed. Herman Buschke designed a 4-minute screening test involving the recall of four items. This test also includes "category cues" to help people remember the items. AD patients are unable to utilize the clues as well as unimpaired adults, so they score lower on the test.

The test procedure is relatively straightforward. The patient is handed a piece of paper with four items printed in large letters and asked to read them aloud. The examiner states each cue, in turn, and the person picks the word that goes with it. For example, if the items are "peach, truck, calculator, shirt," the category cues might be "fruit, vehicle, electronic device, clothing." After a delay of 2 to 3 minutes, during which time the patient is engaged in some other activity, such as counting or drawing, he is asked to recall the items. He gets 2 points for each item he recalls without the cue. He gets 1 point for each item recalled with the cue. If he does not remember the item even with the cue, he gets 0 points. This makes the best possible score 8, and the worst 0. A score of 4 or less is consistent with dementia.

Overall, the memory impairment screen is a simple test that can expose the early memory weakness seen in AD, but it may miss the minority of dementias that present with cognitive problems other than memory as the most afflicted area because of its strict reliance on memory.

> The memory impairment screen is a simple test that can expose the early memory weakness seen in AD.

The Six-Item Screener

Careful analysis of the various items on the MMSE has shown that the ones most sensitive to early AD are the three-word recall and the date.

The six-item screener consists of the three-word recall combined with asking the month, year, and day of the week in between. The patient gets 1 point for each correct item, so scores range from 0 to 6. This test is fast, taking less than a minute to administer. The physician asks the patient to "Repeat and remember these three words: flag, tree, dime." After the person repeats the three words once, the physician asks the patient to state the day, month, and year. Last, the patient is asked to repeat the three words. A score of 3 or less indicates a problem.

In studies so far, the six-item screener has been evaluated primarily in a population dominated by people of lower socioeconomic and educational status, where it was found to be a good tool for distinguishing normal individuals from those with dementia. However, has not been evaluated in a more highly educated sample. By definition, for example, someone with a mild dementia and MMSE scores of 28 or higher will automatically pass the six-item screener.

The Mini-Cog

The mini-cog combines a clock drawing test and a three-item recall test. Soo Borson authored this exam, which is easy to administer and score. It is a pass or fail exam. If the patient recalls all three items, she automatically passes; if she does not recall any of them, she automatically fails. The clock drawing test is used as a tie-breaker in case only one or two items are recalled. If the clock drawing is normal, the patient earns a pass; if not, she earns a fail. The mini-cog has been tested in multiethnic samples and has been shown to significantly improve recognition of both MCI and dementia by primary care doctors. Again, it is not clear how well it performs in the more highly educated population. Because many normal people fail the three-item recall if they are distracted, a failure on either the mini-cog or six-item screener due only to recall should be interpreted cautiously.

The Hopkins Verbal Learning Test

The Hopkins Verbal Learning Test (HVLT) takes about 5 minutes to administer and hence is somewhat longer than the mini-cog and six-item screener. To administer the test, the physician reads a list of twelve words, and immediately afterwards the person repeats as many of them as he can. The procedure is repeated two more times, and the total number of words recalled over the three trials is added up to get the "total recall" score. This is the working memory, immediate recall portion of the test. The physician then reads a list of twenty-four words: the twelve on the original list mixed with twelve new words. The patient is asked to give a "yes" or "no" response for each word as to whether it was on the list. The number of new words the patient claims to remember is subtracted from the number actually recognized as being on the list for the "discrimination index." The total recall score is added to the discrimination index to give the "memory score." Scores range from 12 to 48 with an average range of 30 to 35.

A memory score of less than 25 indicates impairment. This test is better at identifying AD than other dementias because it is restricted to memory. It has not been examined in a mild dementia sample, however.

Dr. D's Quick and Easy (Q & E) Dementia Screening Test

The last dementia screening test discussed here is a relatively new, 2.5 minute exam designed by one of the authors of this book, Paul Dash, who adopted screening tests used by physicians at the University of California at San Diego to create "Dr. D's Q & E." This test is similar to one independently developed by Wes Ashford that is used at the University of Kentucky. The Q & E has four parts, including encoding (learning three paired items; for example: "red ball, white horse, gold key"); temporal orientation (the date); verbal fluency (number of animals named in 1 minute); and recall (pairs). The scoring system for this test is different from other tests because lower scores are better.

For encoding, if the patient repeats the items twice on the first attempt, or with one repetition by the physician, he earns 0 points. If the items must be repeated a second time, he gets 1 point; a third time, 2 points. If he still cannot repeat them all, he is asked to repeat them one by one, thus earning a score of 3. For the temporal orientation portion, patients earn 0 points if they are within 1 day of the date, and 1 point if more than a day off. An additional 2 points are given if they state the wrong month; 3 points if they give the wrong year. For the verbal fluency task, the patient earns 0 points if they name fourteen or more animals, 1 point for ten to thirteen animals, 2 for six to nine animals, 3 for three to five animals, and 4 for zero to two animals. One point is earned if the same animal is repeated two or three times; 2 points are earned if they repeat four or more animals. Finally, for the recall of the three paired items, patients earn one point for every pair missed and a half a point for mixed-up pairs (for example, "red horse").

The scores from each section are added up to arrive at a final Q & E score. Scores range from 0 to 21. A normal score is 0 to 2. Three is a borderline score and scores of 4 or greater typically indicate a problem. The Q & E evaluates more than just memory. Consequently, it may help detect non-AD dementias. This test can also be used to track changes, because it has a relatively large score range. Preliminary research indicates that the Q & E is more sensitive than the MMSE, mini-cog, clock draw, and six-item screener in detecting mild dementia, while still allowing the vast majority of normal people to score within the normal range, regardless of educational background.

> The Q & E is more sensitive than the MMSE, mini-cog, clock draw, and six-item screener in detecting mild dementia.

EXTENSIVE NEUROPSYCHOLOGIC TESTING

Although the dementia screens are useful during office visits, and often provide sufficient information to the doctor, more extensive testing can help diagnose AD and other dementias. Typically, these evaluations are performed by a neuropsychologist. The tests are administered one-on-one, often over the course of 2 or more days in order to minimize fatigue. In-depth testing is necessary in a variety of circumstances. Three common reasons are to rule out illness in the presence of mild or borderline impairment (if the patient's problems are unusual), and when a significant psychiatric history complicates the interpretation of bedside cognitive tests. In any case, tests can be used as a baseline measure so that follow-up exams also include information about changes or the rate of decline.

Specialized tests in multiple cognitive areas can confirm or deny that problems are present and outline their severity if warranted. The neuropsychologist often provides helpful suggestions for utilizing preserved cognitive strengths in problem solving and exercises for improving areas of cognitive weakness. Neuropsychologic testing is also potentially helpful in certain medical/legal situations; for example, when a person's competence to make decisions is at issue.

In AD, there are three tests a patient is likely to encounter that may be portions of a larger comprehensive neuropsychologic battery. The first is the Alzheimer's Disease Association Diagnostic cognition test (ADAS-cog). It takes about 45 minutes to administer, and surveys all aspects of cognition in some detail. The second is the Repeatable Battery for the Assessment of Neuropsychological Status (RBANS). This is a comprehensive test designed for the elderly that takes about a half an hour to administer. Preliminary evidence indicates the RBANS is more sensitive than the MMSE in detecting very mild dementia. Last is the Addenbrooke's Cognitive Examination (ACE) test, developed in England, which also takes about a half-hour to administer. Although these and other tests are readily available, the majority of individuals with a typical history and cognitive evaluation consistent with AD will not require extensive neuropsychologic testing.

STANDARD MEDICAL TESTS FOR DEMENTIA

If the physician discovers significant cognitive problems, either through simple office visit exams or through more extensive neuropsychologic testing, the next step is to try to uncover the potential causes. Blood

> The next step is to try to uncover the potential causes.

41

tests, neuroimaging, electroencephalography (EEG), and the sampling of cerebrospinal fluid (CSF) may all be requested by the doctor.

Blood Tests

The blood tests typically ordered when dementia is suspected include a set of routine tests and some special ones. The routine tests are a complete blood count (CBC) and a comprehensive chemistry panel. The CBC includes tests for the number of white blood cells, which can indicate whether an infection or immunodeficiency syndrome is present, and the hemoglobin and hematocrit, which are measures of the number and size of red blood cells. Changes in red blood cell size may indicate whether certain vitamin or mineral deficiencies are present. For example, iron deficiency causes the red cells to shrink; whereas vitamin B_{12} and folate (folic acid) deficiencies cause them to become enlarged. Last, there is a platelet count. Platelets are involved in blood clotting.

The chemistry panel includes measurement of standard blood chemicals, such as glucose, sodium, potassium, and calcium, as well as the levels of various enzymes and cholesterol. It provides an indication of functioning for certain vital organs, especially the liver and kidneys. The brain requires a healthy level of important minerals and proper functioning of the internal organs in order to work properly. People with untreated liver or kidney failure, or whose blood sugar is too high or too low, will have problems with cognition. Patients often have normal CBC and chemistry panels because disruptions in these systems do not usually accompany AD. In addition to these routine tests, a few special blood tests are recommended. These include measures of thyroid function, usually a serum T4 and thyroid-stimulating hormone (TSH) to check whether the thyroid gland is under- or overactive. Also, vitamin B_{12} and folate levels are checked, as well as the *erythrocyte sedimentation rate* (ESR). The ESR is increased in certain autoimmune diseases, such as *systemic lupus*, which can be associated with cognitive problems. It was formerly recommended that a Venereal Disease Research Laboratory Slide Test (VDRL), a test for syphilis, be routinely ordered, but this is now in the optional category because advanced syphilis affecting the nervous system is very rare these days. In certain areas of the United States where syphilis is highly prevalent, however, this test may still be part of dementia screening. Similar to the routine tests, the specialized blood test results are generally normal in AD patients.

Neurodiagnostic Tests

Just as blood tests are necessary to rule out competing diagnoses, so are tests of brain structure and function. Initially, a physician may order a *computed tomography* (CT) *scan* or *magnetic resonance imaging* (MRI) of the brain. Both studies provide pictures of brain anatomy, and help rule out problems such as brain tumors, strokes, blood clots, or *hydrocephalus* (enlargement of the brain's fluid system). An MRI gives a better overall picture than a CT and is the preferred test, although it is somewhat more expensive. Both tests are safe, but some people with a tendency towards claustrophobia have a difficult time with the MRI. The space in which the head lies is relatively narrow, and occasionally the patient may require a mild sedative. In certain circumstances, the ordering physician may request that the test be performed "with contrast." In this case, the patient is injected with a contrast agent that can improve the visualization of some lesions, such as tumors. Early AD or MCI patients will usually have normal neuroimaging studies, although brain atrophy will be present as the disease progresses (see Chapter 7).

Positron emission tomography (PET) and *single photon emission computed tomography* (SPECT) scans are also sometimes used in dementia diagnosis. Both tests measure metabolic activity in the brain. Of the two, PET shows the brain in more detail, although SPECT is less expensive and more widely available. In AD, both tests show that the temporal and *parietal* areas on both sides of the brain are not as active as in healthy adults. Medicare has indicated that they will now cover PET scans for dementia diagnosis under certain circumstances.

The last neurodiagnostic test that may be requested is the electroencephalogram (EEG), which is a measure of the electrical activity in the brain. During the test, small electrodes are placed on the patient's scalp in order to detect electrical activity generated by neurons in the cortex.

The activity is converted to *waveforms*, which are interpreted by the neurologist. In the waking state, the normal EEG rhythm consists of oscillations in the range of 8 to 13 cycles per second (Hz). The EEG is usually normal in early dementia, but some slowing, typically in the 5 to 7 Hz range, is often seen as the disease progresses. Unfortunately, this type of change is common in many disease states, and it generally does not appear in AD until the dementia is clinically obvious. This prevents the EEG from aiding in an initial dementia diagnosis.

The EEG can be useful for AD in special circumstances. People with AD may experience *seizures*, bursts of electrical activity that disrupt the normal functioning of the brain. Often, an EEG is required to show that this activity is present. Typically, seizures can be treated with an antiepileptic (antiseizure or anticonvulsant) medication.

Lumbar Puncture

A *lumbar puncture* involves insertion of a needle into the lumbar spinal canal to withdraw cerebrospinal fluid (CSF). This diagnostic test is not routinely performed in dementia evaluations. Although quite safe, it is somewhat uncomfortable, and problems with headaches can occur after the procedure. The CSF circulates in and around the brain, and its chemical composition is affected by various brain processes. This test is important in detecting rather rare causes of dementia by infectious agents, such as certain fungi, tuberculosis, and syphilis. In the last several years, however, there has been intense interest in measuring CSF levels of the amyloid and tau proteins as a means of diagnosing AD.

Surprisingly, in AD, the level of CSF amyloid, specifically the Aβ42 peptide, is lower than in normal people, even though more of it is produced in the AD brain (see Chapter 7). The reason given for this is that it is being "swallowed up" by the amyloid plaques and aggregates in the brain so that it does not escape into the CSF. On the other hand, the tau proteins do get into the CSF, so their level is higher in AD patients. The combination of low amyloid and high tau in the CSF is a sensitive and specific marker for AD. This test is commercially available and it is also being used in research.

There has been some debate regarding how valuable the evaluation of the CSF actually is in dementia diagnosis. An experienced neurologist diagnosing AD is right about 85 to 90 percent of the time, as judged by autopsy studies. The CSF test also detects the AD pattern about 90 percent of the time. Presently, the CSF test is not often used in clinical practice, because it is expensive, involves a lumbar puncture, and may have uncomfortable side effects.

In 2001, the American Academy of Neurology published an official *Practice Parameters* consensus paper on dementia diagnosis. They concluded that "there are no CSF or other biomarkers recommended for routine use in determining the diagnosis of AD at this time." The main objection of the AAN to these various tests is that they are not superior to diagnostic accuracy based solely on clinical judgment. In the future, careful studies that validate new procedures and prove the diagnostic value of specific biological or neurodiagnostic tests, will serve to enhance the evaluation of symptoms that may indicate Alzheimer's disease.

Two Tests that May Prove Useful in AD Diagnosis or Treatment

The *neural thread protein* (NTP) has been found in the same areas and in similar densities as neurofibrillary tangles in the AD brain (see Chapter 7). The CSF and urine levels of NTP are also elevated in AD patients. The exact relationship of this protein to AD is not known, but it is under intense investigation. A urine test for NTP is commercially available that detects changes in the amount of NTP in some early AD patients, although this test has not been evaluated with MCI patients.

A second promising test, a blood test, is already widely available. Evidence has shown that an elevated level of *homocysteine*, an amino acid, is a risk factor for AD as well as for cardiovascular disease and stroke. Homocysteine occurs naturally in the body, but at high levels it can cause problems. Homocysteine levels can be affected by dietary levels of vitamins B_6, B_{12}, and folate. Consequently, there are studies investigating whether dietary supplements can lower the risk of AD and vascular disease. Measuring homocysteine levels is not very helpful in diagnosis, however, because normal people can have elevated levels. The B-vitamin supplements that lower homocysteine levels can be considered if homocysteine is elevated.

GENETIC BLOOD TESTS FOR AD

There are blood tests available for genetic mutations responsible for extremely rare cases of AD, and also for a gene that is a risk factor for AD, the ApoE4 allele. These are discussed in more detail in Chapter 12. However, the bottom line is that, at this time, genetic blood tests can be justified only in exceptional circumstances and should not be part of the routine diagnostic evaluation for AD.

SMELL TESTS AND ALZHEIMER'S

Because the entorhinal cortex is frequently involved early in AD (see Chapter 3), and because this area of the brain is important for recognizing smells, a high proportion of people with AD have deficits in this ability. Several studies also indicate that an impaired sense of smell is a risk factor for MCI patients to progress to AD. It has therefore been proposed by some that a standardized test of smell be used as a screening measure. However, because many other common conditions besides dementia can cause smell impairment, such as nasal congestion and prior respiratory infections, and because some studies indicate that reduced smell abilities are present in up to a quarter of the normal elderly population, more study of this proposal is needed before it can be recommended. Therefore the interpretation of the results obtained from various "smell test kits" recently being marketed to the general public for self-diagnostic purposes, must be done with extreme caution. Indeed, with *all* of the test mentioned in this chapter, interpretation by a physician is necessary.

> With *all* of the test mentioned in this chapter, interpretation by a physician is necessary.

Chapter 5

Stages and Prognosis in Alzheimer's

Chapter Question:
How bad is he, and how much
longer does he have?

There is considerable individual variability and, hence, some unpredictability in the course of AD. In general though, the disease is progressive. Chapter 5 explores three commonly used systems to define the stages of Alzheimer's disease and reviews the associated cognitive decline and mortality rates.

THE STAGES OF ALZHEIMER'S DISEASE

A S PATIENTS AND FAMILY MEMBERS learn to cope with AD, they will have important questions about the course of the illness: "What stage is he in?" "Will she get worse?" "How long do we have?" Although there is great individual variation in the course of this disease, physicians can provide some guidelines as to what to expect and when. AD is general-

> There is great individual variation in the
> course of this disease.

ly defined by a progressive worsening of symptoms and loss of function. Breaking the course of a progressive illness into stages is somewhat arbitrary, but still necessary to provide caregivers with some guidance. Several models have been developed, three of which will be described

47

here: the generic "mild-moderate-severe" model, the Clinical Dementia Rating Scale, and the Global Deterioration Scale.

The Generic Model

Although not actually a formal system, the generic classification of patients into mild, moderate, and severe stages is the most commonly used staging system in clinical practice. Often families are told whether the patient is in the mild, moderate, or severe stage simply based on the doctor's intuitive assessment of the situation. Generally speaking, if the person has some obvious cognitive difficulties, but is reasonably communicative and can still accomplish basic self-care and some complex functions, such as using a telephone and household appliances, then she is considered to be in the *mild* phase. Conversely, if the disease has progressed to the point that nursing home placement has occurred or is imminent, she is labeled *severe*. Circumstances in between mild and severe are labeled *moderate*.

To assist in this classification, a physician may use the patient's score from the Mini- Mental Status Examination (MMSE; see Chapter 4). MMSE scores of 20 to 26 are associated with the mild stage of AD; scores of 10 to 19 are associated with the moderate stage; and scores under 10 are associated with the severe stage. MMSE scores do not provide for an exact classification, and other factors should be considered. In addition, as was reviewed in Chapter 4, caution should be used when interpreting the MMSE scores of highly-educated individuals.

The Washington University Clinical Dementia Rating Scale

The Clinical Dementia Rating Scale (CDR) was designed by John Morris. It uses stricter definitions of mild, moderate, and severe dementia than the generic model. Healthy cognition is labeled CDR 0, and questionable cognition is labeled CDR 0.5. A score of 0.5 roughly corresponds to mild cognitive impairment (MCI). The stages of AD are labeled CDR 1 for mild, CDR 2 for moderate, and CDR 3 for severe. Scores are based on the patient's abilities in six domains (Table 5-1). In each domain, the patient

Table 5-1: The Six Domains of the CDR Scale

1. Memory
2. Orientation
3. Judgment and problem solving
4. Community affairs
5. Home and hobbies
6. Personal care

is assigned a score of 0, 0.5 (in some domains), 1, 2, or 3. The average score from the six domains equals the patient's overall CDR score. Typically, the six domains can be assessed in about 40 minutes.

For all domains, a score of 0 represents normal function. In the memory domain, a score of 0.5 indicates mild but consistent forgetfulness. A score of 1 corresponds to moderate memory loss that is worse for recent events; 2 denotes severe memory loss with retention of only highly learned material; and 3 represents only fragmentary memory remaining.

In the orientation domain, people cannot receive a score of 0.5. A CDR score of 1 denotes some difficulty with time relationships; 2 represents disorientation to time and, often, place; and 3 indicates that the patient is oriented to person only.

In the judgment and problem solving domain, a score of 0.5 corresponds to little impairment in solving problems. A score of 1 can be interpreted as a moderate difficulty in handling complex problems but with preserved social judgment; 2 indicates severe impairment in problem solving and impaired social judgment as well; and 3 represents a complete inability to make sound judgments or solve problems.

In the community affairs domain, a CDR score of 0.5 reflects mildly impaired abilities in work, shopping, business, and financial affairs, as well as with social groups. A person scoring 1 requires assistance to function at these activities but may still be engaged in some of them; 2 represents a person who appears well enough to be taken to functions outside of the home, although there is no pretense of independent function; and 3 is given to patients who can no longer be taken to social functions.

In the home and hobbies domain, a 0.5 score reveals a slight impairment in hobbies and intellectual interests. A person scoring 1 shows mild but definite impairment of function at home, with more difficult chores abandoned; 2 corresponds to patients who can perform simple chores, but have poorly sustained and restricted interests. A patient with a 3 in this domain has no ability to function.

Lastly, in the personal care domain, a person cannot receive a 0.5. A CDR score of 1 indicates the person needs some prompting; 2 is given to someone who requires assistance in dressing and hygiene; and finally, a score of 3 corresponds to individuals who require significant aid with personal care and are often incontinent.

Morris provides a summary of strengths and weaknesses for each average overall CDR score:

1. CDR 0.5 (Questionable; MCI): mild forgetfulness; no problems with orientation or personal care; doubtful or mild impairment in judgment, problem solving, and ability to function in the community; and slight impairment in hobbies and interests
2. CDR 1 (mild): moderate memory loss, especially for recent events; some difficulty with time relationships (such as keeping track of the date or month); impaired problem solving abilities; able to maintain interpersonal social judgments (such as smiles and shakes hands appropriately); requires assistance in shopping and financial affairs; has mild but clear impairment in functioning in the home; and requires some prompting for personal care
3. CDR 2 (moderate): severe recent memory loss; not oriented to time (often including the year); severe impairments in judgment and problem solving abilities with some inappropriate social behavior; completely unable to function in the community, although can be taken outside of the home; preservation of ability to do simple chores in the home; and requires assistance with dressing and hygiene
4. CDR 3 (severe): only fragmentary memory function; no idea of time and location; completely unable to solve problems or make appropriate judgments; cannot be taken outside the home; has no ability

to do simple tasks in the home; and requires significant or complete assistance with basic daily living activities.

The patient's CDR score should be evaluated at regular intervals by the physician.

The Global Deterioration Scale

The Global Deterioration Scale (GDS) was developed by B. Reisberg and colleagues and is often used in AD research studies. The GDS uses detailed clinical descriptions of seven major stages, ranging from normal to severe. The clinician reviews symptoms with the patient and caregiver, and then decides which level of severity or stage applies to the patient. Table 5-2 provides an account of what the patient and caregiver can expect as the illness progresses.

Table 5-2: Global Deterioration Scale

Stage 1: No subjective complaints of memory deficit, and none evident on examination

Stage 2: Subjective memory complaints, usually in forgetting names or where objects have been placed

Stage 3: Earliest clear-cut deficits (for example, getting lost, problems retaining information from reading material)

Stage 4: Clear-cut deficit on careful clinical interview (for example, decreased ability to travel and handle finances, decreased knowledge of current events)

Stage 5: Patient can no longer survive without some assistance (for example, cannot recall names of close family members, addresses, or telephone numbers)

Stage 6: May forget name of spouse; largely unaware of all recent events; retains some knowledge of surroundings; delusional behavior and agitation are common in this stage

Stage 7: All verbal abilities and ability to walk lost over the course of this stage; patient is incontinent; motor symptoms such as quick jerking movements (myoclonus) and epileptic seizures can occur in the last two stages

---

RATE OF DECLINE

Pathologically, it often appears that an MCI patient does, in fact, have AD. Many MCI patients remain stable for years, however, and the disease is not always progressive until it reaches the CDR 1 stage, using the clinical dementia rating scale. Most studies suggest that 10 to 20 percent of MCI patients per year convert to mild AD. Decline is inevitable once

> Many MCI patients remain stable for years.

a definite diagnosis of AD is reached. Over two-thirds of mild AD patients will reach the severe stage within 5 years, with the rate of decline often accelerated in the moderate stage. Fortunately, many of the studies predicting this rate of progression were conducted prior to the widespread availability of Alzheimer's medications, which may slow the rate of decline.

Other factors that can have a positive or negative effect on the rate of progression are age at onset, occurrence of behavioral disturbances, motor slowing, and medical illness. Patients who are younger at the age of onset tend to decline faster than those who are older at onset. It is thought that the faster rate in younger patients reflects a more virulent disease process. Patients suffering prominent behavioral disturbances, such as hallucinations, also have a faster rate of decline. Similarly, the presence of parkinsonian-like symptoms, such as motor slowness and stiffness, can signal an accelerated rate of decline. Finally, episodes of significant medical illness are often associated with relatively sudden declines in Alzheimer's patients. As a further complication, AD patients are predisposed to becoming delirious when they are ill for any reason, and often recovery is incomplete. The exact reasons for this are not clear, but a plausible explanation is that some of the relatively fragile connections between the neurons in their brains are disrupted by the co-occurring illness. Once neural communication is interrupted, pathways may become difficult to reestablish.

MORTALITY

In general, the estimated time from the appearance of the first symptoms of AD to the time of death is approximately 5 to 10 years, although the range can be anywhere from 2 to 20 years. Longevity is influenced by gender, the presence of other medical problems, early detection, and the rate of cognitive decline. For example, a study by E.B. Larsen and colleagues at the University of Washington in Seattle estimated a median survival of 4.2 years for men and 5.7 years for women from the time of AD diagnosis. The tendency for women with Alzheimer's to live longer than men occurred in all age groups. People with lower MMSE scores, a tendency to fall, and other medical problems, such as diabetes and heart failure, had shorter life spans. Overall, it is estimated that AD shortens life expectancy by about 5 years. In fact, a paper by J.S. Tschanz from the Cache County study provided evidence that AD had a greater effect on mortality than other chronic diseases, including diabetes and heart disease.

Survival time from diagnosis until death also depends upon how early the diagnosis is made and the rate of cognitive decline. Mortality studies repeatedly report a shorter survival time for those with lower MMSE scores at diagnosis. In addition, a study led by J.S. Hui from Rush Medical Center in Chicago showed that AD patients with the fastest rates of cognitive decline had mortality rates eight times that of those with the slowest rates of decline. These results are similar to those of E.B. Larsen's study, in which individuals whose MMSE scores declined by 5 points or more in 1 year had a 60 percent increase in risk of death.

The journey of the AD patient, family, and friends, although variable in length, will have many similarities. Patients will progress through the stages of illness, each one characterized by less autonomy and more dependence. Caregivers will face new and more difficult challenges. Physicians and researchers will struggle to arrest cognitive decline and

> New medications become available every
> year and small battles are won every day.

reverse the effects of the illness. This predictable pattern of events may seem inevitable, but new medications become available every year and small battles are won every day. We are confident the next decade will provide relief to families living with Alzheimer's and hope to those who are newly diagnosed.

THE PATIENT WHO REFUSES TO SEE THE DOCTOR

The tests mentioned above are well and good, but they are useless if you can't get your loved one in to see the doctor. In Chapter 2, we mentioned the not uncommon situation where family members notice that the person's memory is failing, but he himself denies it. The technical term for this problem of self-awareness is called *anosagnosia*. Patients with anosognosia may see no reason why they should have to see the doctor for what in their view is a nonexistent problem and sometimes may even become paranoid that being taken for a memory evaluation is part of a plot by the family to defraud them. As we will discuss in Chapter 8, such delusions can't be corrected by reasoning with the person. If the person has such a reaction to the mere suggestion of being taken in for an evaluation, it may therefore be a sign that they are already entering the moderate stages of the disease, and hence it becomes all the more critical that they be seen.

So how does one deal with the person who really needs to be seen but who adamantly refuses? In these types of situation, the caregiver often must resort to benign trickery. One strategy is to make the doctor appointment yourself, and shortly before it's time to leave to simply announce that "it's time to get ready for your doctor's appointment for your check-up." Act in a very manner-of-fact way about it. If the patient protests he didn't know about any such appointment, say that the appointment was made a long time ago, and point to your calendar book, where you will have written it in. Explain that at his age regular check-ups are needed for blood pressure, blood tests, and so forth, that the doctor is expecting to see him today and has made room in his appointment schedule for him, will be very disappointed if he doesn't show up, and so forth. Be clear and firm that this doctor visit is going to happen.

A second strategy is to pretend that the doctor visit is for you and request that he accompany you; once you're in the examination room together and the doctor is present, the "switcheroo" can usually be accomplished smoothly. Another idea is to claim that the doctor called and said it was time for an appointment. In any case, the doctor must be informed in advance (and preferably reminded on the day of the visit) that the real purpose of the visit is to evaluate the person's cognitive status.

Chapter 6

Alzheimer's versus Other Causes of Dementia

Chapter Question:
Is it Alzheimer's or something else?

Although Alzheimer's disease is the most common cause of dementia, other causes must be considered when deciding upon a diagnosis. Chapter 6 discusses the reversible dementias, stroke and vascular dementia, dementia with Lewy bodies, fronto-temporal dementia, and *Creutzfeldt-Jakob disease* as other causes of dementia.

REVERSIBLE DEMENTIAS

DOCTORS HAVE A STANDARD PROCESS for diagnosing disease that is uniformly applied to each patient. The first step is to gather information about the person's history from the patient, people who know the patient, and available medical records. This step usually leads to a list of probable disease states. The doctor then examines the patient, paying special attention to signs that should be present or absent in the given disease. The final step includes laboratory tests, imaging studies, and other diagnostic procedures that may further narrow the list of potential diagnoses, or corroborate conclusions based on the history and physical exam.

There is a long list of possible causes of dementia. The most common cause is AD, accounting for about 55 percent of dementia cases. Approximately 15 percent are due solely to stroke, with another 10 percent attributed to a combination of AD and stroke. About 10 percent of dementia cases are caused by Lewy body disease, and 5 percent are attrib-

There is a long list of possible causes of dementia. Alzheimer's disease is a form of dementia.

uted to reversible causes, such as disruptions in metabolism or depression. The remaining 5 percent are the result of miscellaneous neurodegenerative conditions, such as multiple sclerosis. When investigating potential causes, the reversible dementias are considered first, even though they are responsible for only a small proportion of dementia cases. They are fairly easy to rule out because they are typically identifiable through laboratory tests, and they can be alleviated through specific treatments. Table 6-1 lists the common reversible causes of dementia.

Table 6-1: Potentially Reversible Causes of Dementia

1. Vitamin B_{12} deficiency
2. Thyroid disorders
3. Normal pressure hydrocephalus
4. Brain tumors
5. Subdural hematoma
6. Medication and drug effects
7. Metabolic dysfunction
8. Depression
9. Infections of the nervous system

Vitamin B_{12} Deficiency

Vitamin B_{12} deficiency occurs principally in two contexts: 1) strict vegetarians who do not get enough B_{12} in the diet and 2) people with diseases of the gastrointestinal tract, such as pernicious anemia, in which absorption of B_{12} through the gut is disrupted. In addition to cognitive difficulties, people with B_{12} deficiency often develop other neurologic findings, including trouble with nerve endings, which causes sensory loss, and in their spinal cord, which can cause balance problems. Individuals experiencing vitamin deficiencies tend to be relatively young, and, thus, are rarely confused with an AD patient. Nonetheless, there are exceptions to every rule, which is why measuring the serum B_{12} level is part of the routine workup for AD.

On the other hand, patients with dementia may have a coincidental B_{12} deficiency. In these situations, even when the B_{12} deficiency is corrected with supplementation, no change in cognitive function is apparent and patients will continue to decline.

Thyroid Disorders

Thyroid hormones play an important role in metabolism and brain cell maintenance. Hormonal blood levels must be within a certain range in order for the brain to function properly. People with low thyroid function (*hypothyroidism*) become slow cognitively and develop various other symptoms, such as coarse hair, weight gain, and fatigue. People with overactive thyroid function (*hyperthyroidism*) typically suffer from psychiatric symptoms, including anxiety, and physical symptoms, such as a racing heart, tremor, and weight loss. Although they usually do not develop a dementia, there have been rare cases of documented dementia with hyperthyroidism where the dementia reversed with treatment. In practice, it is very rare for hypothyroidism to be a cause for dementia. In a study with over 2,700 hypothyroid patients, only one presented with dementia that reversed with treatment. There is substantial evidence, however, that people with low thyroid function—although perhaps not demented—score more poorly on cognitive tests than those with normal function, and that such cognitive problems are reversible with treatment. In addition, people with low thyroid function feel much better when they take thyroid supplements.

A *serum thyroid stimulating hormone* (TSH) level and a T4 (thyroid hormone with four iodine atoms attached) are usually adequate to check for thyroid problems. These studies are usually routinely done as part of a dementia evaluation.

Normal Pressure Hydrocephalus

Normal pressure hydrocephalus (NPH) is characterized by an expansion of the *ventricles* in the brain, which contain cerebrospinal fluid (CSF).

CSF is created as a filtrate from the blood by special cells in the ventricles called the *choroid plexus*. CSF circulates through the ventricles, down into the spinal canal, and is absorbed into the brain. It is this absorption process that becomes partially blocked in NPH, resulting in a buildup of CSF. Clinically there are three main symptoms: dementia, urinary incontinence, and balance disturbance. Brain imaging reveals that the ventricles are greatly enlarged; whereas any shrinkage of the cerebral cortex is minimal by contrast. A lumbar puncture is often performed for diagnostic purposes, revealing that the CSF pressure is normal, hence the name.

Treatment involves the placement of a shunt tube into the ventricles to drain the accumulated CSF. This can result in dramatic improvement, at least in the short term, although the shunt may develop various problems in the long term, such as infection. A brain biopsy can be done conveniently at the time of shunt placement. This involves taking a tiny piece of cortex to study under the microscope. The tissue will be examined for the characteristic AD pathology of plaques and tangles (see Chapter 7). Thus, the patient's response to the shunt and the results of the biopsy can be used to definitively identify the cause of the dementia. People with more prominent balance problems tend to respond better to shunt placement than those who have more prominent dementia.

Brain Tumors

Brain tumors are a potentially treatable, although uncommon cause of dementia. Usually a person with a tumor will have symptoms besides changes in cognition that indicate the illness is not due to AD. Often the patient will experience weakness or sensory loss on the side opposite the lesion. The diagnosis of a brain tumor is immediately clear upon viewing the neuroimaging.

Treatment and prognosis depend upon the type of tumor, its location, and operability. For example, a *meningioma* is a slow growing benign tumor that compresses the brain from the outside. Removal is often curative. A small nonsymptomatic meningioma discovered by chance with imaging may not even warrant treatment, except for follow-up imaging every 1 to 2 years. On the other hand, a *glioblastoma* is a malignant tumor that grows within the substance of the brain. Treatment nearly always has, at most, a temporary effect. Prognosis is poor, even in young people, and may signal an untimely death in the elderly, usually within a few months. Finally, the most common type of brain tumor is *metastatic* cancer, usually from the lung or, in women, the breast. This results in several brain sites where the cancer cells have taken hold and grown. Radiation and chemotherapy can provide some benefit, although they are ordinarily not curative. On occasion, if only one metastatic lesion is present, surgery can be performed.

Subdural Hematoma

A *subdural hematoma* is a blood clot that produces symptoms by compressing the brain. It is often caused by a blow to the head, although in the elderly the trauma may be minor. In some instances, the blow may not even be recalled, or may have been dismissed as trivial for example, banging the head against a door. An imaging study is diagnostic, and in this case *computed tomography* (CT) is better than *magnetic resonance imaging* (MRI). The treatment is often curative, and involves a neurosurgeon drilling a hole in the skull to drain the blood clot. Small subdural hematomas, especially if they are too small to drain, may simply be watched for signs of progression. Large subdural hematomas are often fatal, especially if the trauma was severe enough to cause other types of brain injury.

Medication and the Effects of Drugs

The effects of medication are a more common reversible cause for cognitive problems in the elderly. Many elderly patients take several medications regularly, so problems with drug interactions can be frequent. Sometimes, even if the patient also suffers from AD, elimination or a change in certain medications can be helpful. Three medications that can cause memory problems, and that are often used among aging patients, are medications that have *anticholinergic* side effects (see Chapter 3), nar-

> The effects of medication are a common reversible cause for cognitive problems in the elderly.

cotics, and sedatives. Table 6-2 lists some common medications that can have cognitive side effects. This table is by no means exhaustive and consultation with a physician or pharmacist is recommended.

Table 6.2: Medications with Cognitive Side Effects

Anticholinergic:
amitriptyline (Elavil®), diphenhydramine (Benadryl®), benztropine (Cogentin®), doxepin (Adapin®), imipramine (Tofranil®), nortriptyline (Pamelor®), oxybutynin (Ditropan®), paroxetine (Paxil®), thioridazine (Mellaril®)

Narcotics:
codeine (in Tylenol 3®), hydrocodone (in Vicodin®), oxycodone (in Percocet® and Percodan®)

Sedatives/Anxiolytics:
alprazolam (Xanax®), lorazepam (Ativan®), diazepam (Valium®), butalbital (such as Fioricet®), alchohol

Some nonprescription drugs, especially the older antihistamines, such as diphenhydramine (Benadryl®), have prominent anticholinergic side effects. Medications such as oxybutynin (Ditropan®), which are used for controlling incontinence, have documented cognitive side effects. The older generation of *tricyclic antidepressant* agents (including amitriptyline [Elavil®]), has prominent anticholinergic action. Painkillers, including codeine or hydrocodone, can have a marked effect on cognition in the elderly (commonly used products are Tylenol 3® and Vicodin®). Last, sedatives and anxiolytics (antianxiety drugs), such as diazepam (Valium®), alprazolam (Xanax®), and alcohol, are also potential culprits in causing compromised cognition in the elderly.

An article by B.H. Mulsant and colleagues highlights the importance of drugs and cognition in the elderly. They measured serum anticholinergic activity in 201 randomly selected elderly patients from the community and correlated the results with MMSE (Mini-Mental

Status Examination) scores. They found at least some anticholinergic activity in 90 percent of the volunteers. Those with higher levels of anticholinergic activity had lower scores on the MMSE. Although tests of anticholinergic activity are not available for routine clinical use, they may become part of the routine workup for dementia in the elderly.

A special word should be added here about alcoholism in the elderly. Obviously, being both old and inebriated is not good for your thinking abilities, and it takes less alcohol to affect cognition in the elderly than in younger people. So, although a glass or two of wine at dinner a few times a week is not a problem, and, in fact, as discussed in the chapter on risk factors, may even help prevent AD, daily consumption of more than a limited amount can be at the root of an apparent dementia. A vigilant eye needs to be kept, particularly on those who have a history of problem drinking earlier in life. When used in combination with certain medications, however, it can exacerbate side effects. Drug abuse is not a common problem in the elderly—most drug abusers either die young or quit—but if this is suspected, a urine toxicology screen is appropriate.

Metabolic Dysfunction

Metabolic causes of cognitive problems are also common in the elderly, although ordinarily they are more associated with acute medical illness than with diseases such as AD. *Metabolic* refers to changes in body chemistries that are generally the result of problems in internal organs. For example, patients with chronic kidney failure who require the use of dialysis are at risk for cognitive impairment. Slowed cognition is also common in people with advanced liver disease, because the liver is unable to detoxify the compounds that can affect thinking. People with advanced lung disease will have difficulty thinking if they cannot get enough oxygen into their blood, or if the levels of carbon dioxide get dangerously high. These metabolic problems are generally quickly detected from the history and routine laboratory tests.

Depression

Depression is related to AD in three important ways:

1. The rate of depression is higher among AD patients than among nondemented adults.
2. Having a depressive episode is associated with an increased risk for developing AD.
3. Depressive symptoms can be confused with dementia in older adults.

> Depressive symptoms can be confused with dementia in older adults.

Effective treatment depends upon the accurate distinction of depressive symptoms and similar symptoms attributed to AD. Chapter 8 discusses the symptoms, diagnosis, and treatment of depression.

Infections of the Nervous System

Infections of the brain usually cause a rapid change in the person's level of awareness, along with focal neurologic signs (for example, paralysis), so they are rarely confused with AD. However, certain uncommon infections of the nervous system with fungal organisms can occasionally produce an AD-like picture that can be treated with special antibiotics. Additionally, the HIV virus can produce a dementia, although there are very few patients with AIDS who are elderly. This may change as new treatments prolong their lives. Advanced syphilis was the most common cause of dementia a century ago, but it is now treatable with penicillin. A lumbar puncture can be done in suspicious cases to check for various infections. Blood tests for HIV and syphilis are readily available.

How Common Are Reversible Dementias?

How common are reversible dementias, and how often do they truly reverse? The news is not encouraging. Dr. A. Mark Clarfield surveyed the literature on this subject in 1988, and again in 2003. He reviewed thirty-nine articles that looked at the prevalence of different kinds of dementia. After combining the results of these studies, he found that only 9 percent of 5,620 dementia cases were potentially reversible, and only 0.6 percent of them actually showed some degree of reversal; just half of these fully reversed. In other words, of the 5,620 cases, only eighteen were cured. This actual rate of reversal is much lower than what has been optimistically estimated by various authorities as accounting for up to 30 percent of dementia cases.

STROKE AND ALZHEIMER'S DISEASE

The relationship of cerebrovascular disease to AD and dementia is a widely researched area. There are several types of strokes, also known as *cerebrovascular accidents* (CVA). The most common CVA is caused by a blockage in a brain artery, resulting in the death of the brain tissue supplied by that artery. This kind of stroke is referred to as an *ischemic* stroke. Less commonly, a stroke results from a ruptured blood vessel, with consequent leakage of blood into the brain. This type of stroke is called a *hemorrhagic* stroke. Symptoms of either type of stroke depend upon the location and extent of the brain area damaged. There are many risk factors for stroke, including smoking, hypertension, diabetes, high cholesterol, a history of heart attack and certain irregular heart rhythms, and a family history of stroke. *Atherosclerosis*, or what is colloquially referred to as "hardening of the arteries," is a major cause of ischemic stroke and results from a complex interplay of the various risk factors.

Some cases of dementia from stroke, or *vascular dementia*, are obvious; for example, the person has a history of one or more debilitating strokes accompanied by clear neurologic symptoms, such as weakness on one side and an imaging study showing big holes, or infarcts, in the brain. This type of dementia from stroke is also called *cortical dementia*. Other types of vascular dementia can result from a relatively small stroke that is located in a particularly vital area; this is called a *strategic infarct dementia*. Multiple small strokes can also add up and cause dementia, or a person can have a combination of small and large strokes.

The result of some strokes is not so obvious. Some strokes do not even cause overt symptoms. These very small strokes can be visualized on MRI scans. The relative importance of these events can be difficult to determine. Although having a small number of *microvascular infarcts* does not produce noticeable cognitive problems, larger numbers are associated with problems in several areas, mainly with general processing speed and executive function (e.g., decision-making ability, judgment, ability to plan ahead, and mental flexibility). Generally, older age and increased severity of vascular risk factors are associated with higher numbers of these lesions. Last, people with AD who also have large numbers of microvascular infarcts tend to be worse off than those without such lesions (see below).

Stroke, while it clearly does not guarantee dementia, is an overall risk factor for developing vascular dementia and even AD. A study by Larry Honig and colleagues estimated that people with stroke have a 50 percent greater chance of developing AD, particularly if they have vascular risk factors. They also tend to develop AD at a younger age, as compared with older people who have not had a stroke. Although the risk is apparent, it is unclear if the brain damage is simply additive or if there is some mechanism by which stroke actually enhances the AD process.

Vascular Dementia

The formal diagnosis of a vascular dementia can be tricky. The gold standard is a brain autopsy, especially since that is the only way that the possibility of concurrent AD can be ruled in or out. Clinically, there are several recommended diagnostic strategies. The criteria rely on various combinations of the following three factors:

1. Clinical stroke temporally related to dementia (for example, the person has a diagnosed stroke and within 3 months also develops dementia symptoms)
2. Critical lesions on neuroimaging
3. Focal findings on neurologic examination, such as weakness or sensory loss on one side or changes in reflexes

A study by David Knopman and colleagues reviewed the autopsy data on dementia patients and compared the results with how well the different definitions were able to identify the vascular dementia cases. Of the 419 patients, half the cases were caused by AD; one-fourth had vascular disease; and the remaining one-fourth had other types of dementia. Only about half of the patients with vascular dementia (12 percent of the total) had pure vascular dementia, the rest also had AD pathology. The researchers found that, overall, the Mayo clinic criteria provided the best classification process. Their criteria simply includes fulfillment of either number 1 (temporal relationship) or number 2 (lesions on neuroimaging), as outlined above.

The relationship between stroke and AD remains complex. There are several types of stroke that vary in their effects depending on number, size, and location of the lesions. Stroke can make the deficits of AD worse

> The relationship between stroke and AD remains complex.

and possibly increase the chances of developing AD. Some dementia patients will have both stroke and AD, whereas others may have purely vascular dementia. Differential diagnosis depends upon the criteria used by the physician and the number and degree of overt symptoms.

What Do the Small Strokes Seen on MRI Mean?

Many strokes do not cause overt symptoms. These very small strokes are often referred to as *microvascular infarcts* or *deep white matter disease*, because they tend to be located not in the cerebral cortex, or gray matter, but in the white matter underneath the cortex. They are frequently visualized on MRI scans. A common clinical situation is for a doctor to order an MRI scan on a patient with cognitive problems and get back a report stating the patient has had this type of small stroke. Often, both the doctor and the family are not sure what to make of these results. There is, in fact, great controversy over what role these small, asymptomatic strokes play in cognitive functioning. Research supports the following four conclusions regarding these lesions:

1. Although a small number of microvascular infarcts does not produce a detectable amount of cognitive problems, larger numbers of them are associated with cognitive problems in a number of areas, mainly having to do with executive function and general processing speed.
2. The number of these lesions is a function of age and the number and severity of vascular risk factors, with hypertension and diabetes probably the most important.
3. Microvascular lesions are an important cause of problems with balance and gait in the elderly (the work of Dr. Robert Baloh at UCLA has been particularly significant on this point).
4. People with AD who have larger amounts of microvascular disease tend to be worse off than those without such lesions.

DEMENTIA WITH LEWY BODIES

Dementia with Lewy bodies (DLB) was first described in 1984, by Larry Hansen at the University of California at San Diego. Lewy bodies are pathologic structures found inside some brain cells in patients with DLB or Parkinson's disease. In Parkinson's disease, Lewy bodies are generally restricted to just a few brain areas, but in DLB they are scattered throughout the brain, including the cerebral cortex and hippocampus. Estimates of the frequency of DLB range from 5 to 20 percent of patients with dementia. DLB can occur as a pure disease or mixed with AD pathology. The exact relationship between the Lewy bodies and the plaques and tangles associated with AD in these latter cases is not clear. Their co-occurrence could be coincidental, but some scientists suspect that a common process underlies both of them.

Clinically, DLB patients have a dementia that is characterized by prominent visual hallucinations, day-to-day fluctuations in functioning, parkinsonian-like features, including slowness of movement and a certain type of muscle stiffness, and sometimes REM behavior disorder. The normal paralysis seen in REM sleep (the dreaming stage) is absent in

REM behavior disorder, so patients physically act out their dreams, sometimes resulting in injury. The distinction between DLB and AD can be difficult, because AD patients can have hallucinations, particularly in the moderate stage. Parkinsonian-like symptoms can also be common in the moderate to advanced AD patient. Fluctuations in day-to-day functioning can provide a crucial difference between the two dementias. Table 6-3 lists four components of these fluctuations. According to T. J. Ferman and colleagues, a "yes" response to three or four of these components readily distinguishes DLB from AD.

DLB can be distinguished from the dementia that often accompanies Parkinson's disease by its time course. In true Parkinson's, the patient has motor problems for many years before the dementia, whereas dementia is an early feature of DLB. DLB patients are susceptible to having severe adverse reactions to the older generation antipsychotic medications, such as haloperidol (Haldol®). DLB patients respond well to the same medications used for AD and parkinsonian-like symptoms, and will often show some response to the medications used to treat Parkinson's disease, such as levodopa.

Table 6-3: Four Components of Fluctuations In DLB

1. Is the patient drowsy or lethargic all the time, or several times per day, despite getting enough sleep the night before?
2. Does the patient spend more that 2 hours sleeping during the day (before 7:00 p.m.)?
3. Does the patient stare into space for long periods of time?
4. Are there times when the patient's flow of ideas seems disorganized, unclear, or illogical?

FRONTOTEMPORAL DEMENTIAS

Several pathologic types of frontotemporal dementia (FTD) share the same basic clinical characteristics. These include an early and progressive change in personality, loss of insight, reduced concern and empathy, a tendency to become slovenly, and the development of odd food cravings, especially for sweets. These personality and lifestyle changes often lead to marital discord and psychiatric referral. Consequently, it is not uncommon for a FTD patient to be misdiagnosed as depressed.

Clinically, FTD can be distinguished from AD by relative preservation of memory, although MRI and PET scans show disproportionate frontal and temporal atrophy or hypometabolism, respectively. Occasionally, FTD is accompanied by progressive motor weakness, which is a type of amyotrophic lateral sclerosis (Lou Gehrig's disease). FTD does not respond to AD medications and treatment is generally unsatisfactory.

A rare variant of FTD is *primary progressive aphasia*. These patients selectively lose their language abilities before they lose other cognitive functions. They are occasionally confused with AD patients, who also manifest language difficulties, but these FTD patients have preserved memory function early in the illness; whereas in AD, memory is often significantly compromised before a language disturbance becomes clinically apparent.

CREUTZFELDT-JAKOB DISEASE

Creutzfeldt-Jakob disease (CJD) is a very rare, ordinarily rapidly progressive dementia syndrome. Patients are usually dead within 3 to 6 months of symptom onset, although occasionally longer survival is possible. Besides the rapid progression, the disease distinguishes itself from AD by the development of uncontrollable muscle jerks called *myoclonus*. The presence of myoclonus usually prompts the ordering of an EEG, which will likely show a characteristic, highly abnormal brain wave pattern. In addition, a test of cerebrospinal fluid (CSF) will likely reveal the 14-3-3 protein; often considered diagnostic of CJD. A form of CJD in animals is "mad cow disease," which has received enormous media attention because of the risk of contracting the disease by eating infected meat. The biology of CJD, which involves a type of protein, or prion, that can be both infectious and inherited has attracted intense scientific interest and resulted in one of the pioneering researchers in this field, Dr. Stanley Prusiner of UCSF, receiving the Nobel Prize in 1997 for his work. As of this writing, there is no effective treatment for CJD or its variants.

CONCLUDING REMARKS

Alzheimer's disease may be the most common cause of dementia, but it is certainly not the only cause. A physician should be consulted imme-

> Early intervention is the best hope for treatment.

diately if symptoms of dementia are noticed in a loved one. The source of the problem must be identified in order for the patient to receive the appropriate treatment. Some causes can be reversed, while the progress of others can only be slowed. Regardless of the cause, early intervention is the best hope for treatment.

Chapter 7

Anatomy and Biochemistry in Alzheimer's

Chapter Question:
What exactly is going on in the brain
of an Alzheimer's patient?

This chapter reviews the characteristic anatomical markers of
AD, including brain atrophy and the presence of amyloid
plaques and neurofibrillary tangles.

THE APPEARANCE OF THE BRAIN

AD IS A DISEASE SPECIFICALLY OF THE BRAIN. This means that although
brain appearance and function are distorted in AD, the rest of the
body appears normal. It is very common to see an elderly patient who is
the picture of physical health, who sees doctors only rarely for routine
check-ups, takes no medications, has normal blood pressure, and walks
in with a spry gait, but who cannot remember a thing!

The most striking abnormality in AD is the appearance of the brain.
For example, compare the appearance of a normal brain to that of an
atrophied AD brain in Figure 7-1. The amount of brain substance in the
folds on the surface of the brain (called *gyri*) is much less in the AD
brain, and the spaces between the folds (called *sulci*) are grossly
enlarged. The *cerebral cortex*—the outer surface of the brain, which is critical to all of our intellectual abilities—has shrunken to a shadow of its
former self. This shrinkage is called *atrophy*. This term may appear as a

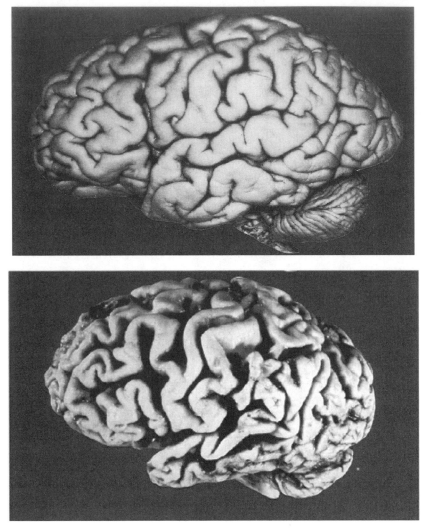

FIGURE 7-1

Normal brain (top) and AD brain (bottom). The front of the brain is to the left. Note the profound thinning of the folds of the AD brain (atrophy), with relative sparing of the back of the brain. (Photos courtesy of Dr. Jody Carey-Bloom, UC San Diego.)

descriptor of the brain, for example, in the report of a MRI scan of a patient with AD.

After documenting this obvious deviation from normal, the next logical step is to question why there is such remarkable shrinkage. The first stage in this process involves a detailed, microscopic examination of a brain (taken at autopsy) prepared with dyes that stain, or highlight, the tissues of interest. Different tissues may be highlighted depending upon which staining procedure is used. For example, some stains highlight random individual nerve cells in the brain, which are called *neurons** (*Golgi stain*), others highlight the nuclei of all the cells (*Nissl stain*), and still others highlight just the white matter of the brain (*myelin stain*). Two of the most critical stains in relationship to AD are the *Congo red stain* and the *silver stain*. These bring out the two central hallmarks seen in the Alzheimer's brain: the *amyloid plaque* and the *neurofibrillary tangle* (Figure 7-2 and 7-3).

> The two central hallmarks seen in the Alzheimer's brain are the *amyloid plaque* and the *neurofibrillary tangle.*

The amyloid plaques seen in these are found outside of neurons. The neurofibrillary tangles are found inside of neurons. The neurofibrillary tangles fill the brain cells until they eventually die. The brains of AD patients are full of these two types of lesions, and together they cause death and shrinkage of neurons, which in turn leads to the atrophy we see in the whole brain (Figure 7-1). Understanding the details of what causes these formations is critical to understanding the causes of AD. Consequently, the next stage in the process of determining the cause of atrophy is to investigate why AD brains get such pathologic formations.

Amyloid Plaques

Over the years, a close examination of amyloid plaques has revealed the details of their form and function. These plaques are composed mainly of a protein that is called the β-*amyloid protein*. It is actually a small fragment of

---

*Besides neurons—the brain cells responsible for information processing—another cell type in the brain, called *glia*, plays a critical support role for the neurons. *Oligodendroglia* wrap the neurons in a *myelin sheath*, which improves their electrical conductivity; *astroglia* play various nutritional and metabolic roles; and *microglia* are involved in inflammatory reactions.

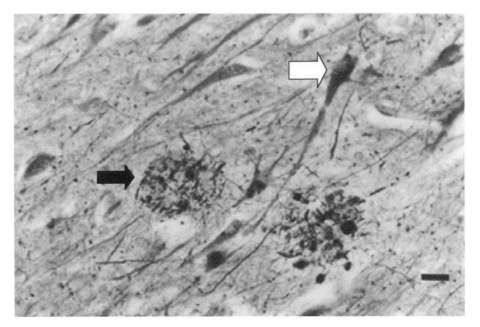

FIGURE 7-2

Silver stain of AD brain. The irregular circular blobs are the amyloid plaques (dark arrow). Neurofibrillary tangles inside of a neuron take up the silver stain, turning it dark (white arrow).

a much larger protein, the *amyloid precursor protein,* or "APP" for short. Like all proteins, the APP is made up of a string of amino acids, 770 of them to be exact. The APP protein lives in normal brain cell membranes (the covering of the cell), although exactly what it does is not clear at this time. Like most proteins, it is created inside the cell, transported to where it is supposed to go (in this case the cell membrane), and after a time it is broken down. There are two major pathways for this breakdown (Figure 7-4). One is a pathway commonly used in normal cells, but the second pathway results in the abnormal processes documented in AD and other dementias.

In the first, normal pathway, the APP is split initially by an enzyme called α-secretase*, and then further by β-secretase. The fragments pro-

---

*α is the first letter of the Greek alphabet, and is pronounced alpha. β pronounced beta, is the second letter, and γ (gamma) is the third.

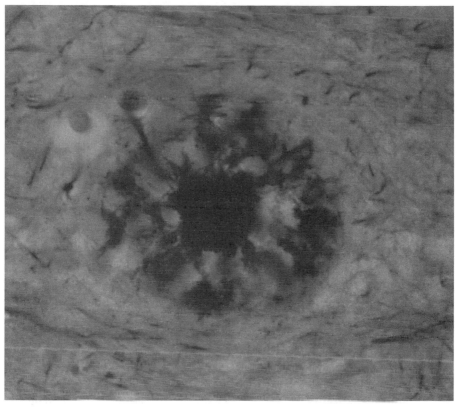

FIGURE 7-3

Higher magnification view of the microscopic pathology of the AD brain. A large amyloid plaque is seen in the center of the picture. The fine dark threads represent neurofibrillary tangles. Bielchowsky silver stain; photo courtesy of Kenneth B. Fallon, M.D., LSU Health Sciences Center-New Orleans, Department of Pathology.

duced are harmless. In the second, abnormal pathway, the APP is split initially by an enzyme called β-secretase, and then by the γ-secretase. These fragments consist of 40 or 42 amino acid length fragments, or *peptides*, which are called the amyloid beta 40 (Aβ40) or amyloid beta 42 (Aβ42) peptides. Several Aβ42 peptides may stick together, forming a short chain, or *oligomer*. Recently these oligomers have also been termed ADDL for *amyloid-beta derived diffusible ligands*, and are the target of new diagnostic and therapeutic interventions (see Chapter 16). Oligomers of Aβ42 have been shown to disrupt communication between neurons.

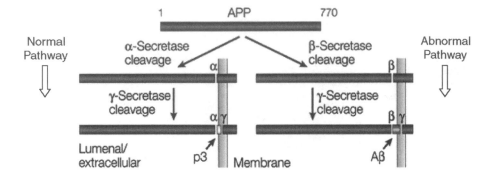

Nature Reviews | Molecular Cell Biology

FIGURE 7-4

Pathways of APP breakdown.

Furthermore, larger amounts of Aβ42, when stuck together, form tiny fibers, called *fibrils*, which stick together to form an amyloid plaque. They can also form small circles, or pores, which may insert themselves into the neuron cell membrane. This results in various substances outside the cell getting inside the cell and causing problems. Therefore, the balance between the two amyloid pathways—the healthy αγ pathway and the pathologic βγ pathway—determines whether a person stays healthy or develops AD. Any factor that tips APP processing towards the βγ pathway is potentially damaging, because it results in a buildup of the Aβ42 peptide and subsequent neuronal dysfunction and death. Interestingly, the balance between the two pathways seems to be affected by the amount of cholesterol in the cell membrane, with lower cholesterol concentrations favoring the αγ pathway. Consequently, certain drugs that affect cholesterol levels may prove to play a role in AD treatment.

Neurofibrillary Tangles (NFT)

The second major pathologic finding in AD brains are the neurofibrillary tangles, which are composed of a different protein called *tau protein*. In the ordinary neuron, tau proteins are found attached to structures called *microtubules*, a crucial part of the "skeleton" of the neuron. In AD, these proteins become *hyperphosphorylated*—meaning they bind extra phosphate groups. This process results from overactive enzymes, called *kinases*, which are responsible for normal phosphate attachment. The byproduct of this overactive process may be that groups of hyperphosphorylated proteins stick together to form helical structures, called *paired helical filaments*. These filaments form the neurofibrillary tangles seen in Figures 7-2 and 7-3 that eventually result in cell death.

Although most AD patients show evidence of amyloid plaques and neurofibrillary tangles, a small subset appear to have "plaque-only" pathology. These patients tend to have a more gradual rate of deterioration than those who have the dual pathology of amyloid and neurofibrillary tangles. On the other hand, patients who have only neurofibrillary tangles are often diagnosed with frontotemporal dementia. Consequently, although protein mutation alone can eventually lead to some type of dementia, it is the co-occurrence of these formations in AD patients that has become the focus of the investigation as to the causes of AD.

Although a complete explanation of the relationship between amyloid plaques and neurofibrillary tangles with respect to AD has not yet been achieved, there is some evidence that the location and timing of these formations may be critical. For example, there is a closer correlation between the location of neurofibrillary tangles in the brains of AD patients and their symptoms than between the location of plaques and symptoms. The tangles first appear in the parts of the brain involved in memory formation (the hippocampus and entorhinal cortex); whereas amyloid plaques are not found there in high concentrations until later in the disease. Yet, there is evidence that $A\beta42$ can accelerate NFT formation. It may be that the small oligomers of $A\beta42$ trigger NFT formation, and only later do the deposits of $A\beta42$ become sufficiently large enough to form amyloid plaques.

UNANSWERED QUESTIONS

To briefly review, the most profound physical result of Alzheimer's disease is brain shrinkage caused by neuronal death. The neurons die as a

> The most profound physical result of
> Alzheimer's disease is brain shrinkage caused
> by neuronal death.

result of the cumulative effects of the two major lesions seen in AD: amyloid deposition and formation of neurofibrillary tangles. Both pathologies result from the abnormal processing of proteins in the brain, although the exact nature of their relationship to one another is a matter of active research.

The scientific community is aggressively researching the unanswered questions, such as:

- Why does the AD process start in one area of the brain as compared to another?
- Why does it spread in a particular pattern?
- Why are some areas, including the primary motor, sensory, and visual cortex, spared until very late in the disease?

One speculative theory under investigation is that the neurons in the brain's memory centers are the most susceptible to the effects of β-amyloid, but that once abnormal processes begin there, a chain reaction is initiated that can spread to other, less susceptible, neurons. Although many questions regarding the biological explanation of Alzheimer's disease remain elusive at this time, the simple facts regarding the location and timing of the pathologic processes help to clarify the pattern and development of the clinical behaviors of those with AD.

Chapter 8

Alzheimer's, Depression, and Other Neuropsychiatric Symptoms

Chapter Question:
Is her thinking muddled because she's depressed?

The relationship between depression and Alzheimer's disease is complex. Depression can be a risk-factor for AD, a result of AD, confused with AD, or be completely unrelated to AD. Effective treatment depends upon the accurate distinction of depressive symptoms and similar symptoms attributed to AD. Other neuropsychiatric symptoms are also likely to occur and should be reviewed by a physician.

DIAGNOSING DEPRESSION

A DIAGNOSIS OF DEPRESSION is based upon the clinical history given by the patient and, in some cases, the caregiver. *The Diagnostic and Statistical Manual of Mental Disorders, 4th Edition* (DSM-IV), outlines the diagnostic criteria, commonly associated behaviors, and detailed descriptions of all identified psychiatric illnesses. Depression typically includes

> Depression typically includes mood, appetite, sleep, and cognitive changes.

Table 8-1: DSM-IV Criteria for a Major Depressive Episode

The person must have at least five of the following symptoms for a period of 2 weeks or longer:

1. Depressed mood
2. Markedly diminished interest or pleasure in activities
3. Significant weight loss or loss of appetite
4. Insomnia (trouble falling asleep) or hypersomnia (too much sleep)
5. Psychomotor retardation or agitation (motor slowing or restlessness)
6. Loss of energy
7. Feelings of worthlessness or guilt
8. Decreased ability to concentrate
9. Recurrent thoughts of death or suicide

At least one of these symptoms must be depressed mood that lasts most of the day nearly every day, or markedly diminished interest or pleasure in all, or almost all, daily activities nearly every day. Symptoms cannot be better explained by bereavement, drug abuse, or a medical condition.

mood, appetite, sleep, and cognitive changes. Symptoms can interfere with work or family responsibilities, and treatment may involve therapy, medication, or both. Table 8-1 contains the DSM-IV criteria for Major Depressive Episode. The last sentence in Table 8-1 includes the exclusion of a medical disorder that may account for the symptoms. This criterion may complicate the diagnosis of depression in AD patients.

DEPRESSION IN ALZHEIMER'S DISEASE

Depression is related to AD in three important ways:

- There are higher rates of depression among AD patients than among nondemented adults.
- Having a depressive episode is associated with an increased risk for developing AD.
- Depressive symptoms can be confused with dementia in older adults.

A further complication of these relationships is that doctors cannot always rely on the patient to give an accurate history, so caregivers should be available to help with symptom reporting and the time course.

Rates of Depression in AD

The Cardiovascular Health Study included a measure of neuropsychiatric symptoms. The authors found that one-third of the 362 dementia patients and one-fifth of the 320 patients with mild cognitive impairment (MCI) had experienced symptoms of depression in the month prior to their interview. The incidence of depression in each sample was significantly greater than that for normal adults.

Similar findings were reported by the Multi-Institutional Research in Alzheimer's Genetic Epidemiology (MIRAGE) study. Although this study was not focused on depression in AD, researchers did ask two important questions. All of the patients and some of the nondemented family members were asked if they had experienced any depressive symptoms that were sufficient to interfere with social and occupational functions, and if they had, how old were they when it happened. A "yes" response certainly was not diagnostic of depression, but it did indicate that the person felt impaired by their depressive symptoms. The investigators found that AD patients were twice as likely as family members to answer in the affirmative.

Depression and the Risk of Developing AD

The MIRAGE study also noted the age at which depressive symptoms were experienced, and compared ages and symptoms within families. In the year before the patient was diagnosed with AD, the patient was four-and-a-half times as likely as family members to experience depressive symptoms. At 10 years and over 25 years prior to the AD diagnosis, patients were still 1.7 times as likely as family members to have experienced depressive symptoms. The authors concluded that depressive symptoms may be a risk factor for later development of AD.

A second study, led by Wilson, came to the same conclusion. This study followed 821, over-65, Catholic clergy members for 7 years. At the first evaluation, participants reported an average of one depressive symptom from a list of ten, but all were cognitively normal at the start of the study. After 7 years, 108 members had developed AD. When the number of depressive symptoms was correlated with the risk of developing AD and the rate of cognitive decline, researchers found that for each depressive symptom endorsed, the risk of developing AD increased by about 20 percent, and the decline in cognition increased by about 25 percent. In addition, those with higher initial depressive symptom scores had a greater risk of developing AD.

Depression and Pseudodementia

Depression may go undiagnosed because of symptoms that are similar to AD. There is also the risk of depression in an elderly person being misdiagnosed as AD. When patients who appear to have AD but, in fact, have only depression, they are said to have *depressive pseudodementia.*

> Depression may go undiagnosed because of symptoms that are similar to AD.

Depressive pseudodementia patients are different from depressed-only and AD-only patients. Depression can result in problems performing cognitive tasks, especially with attention and memory. Depressed pseudodementia patients meet all of the criteria for depression, but on cognitive testing they resemble AD patients. They do not meet the other requirements for an AD diagnosis, however. Unfortunately, this can make the diagnosis of depressive pseudodementia problematic. Some studies of brain metabolism using SPECT scans in patients diagnosed with depressive pseudodementia show a pattern of abnormalities more similar to AD patients than patients with depression only (see Chapter 4).

It is generally recommended that all elderly patients with depression be evaluated for cognitive decline at regular intervals. Likewise, patients with AD should be regularly evaluated for depression. Depressive pseudodementia patients may need to be evaluated more often, however, because their diagnosis may be a warning that they will develop AD relatively soon.

Depression in Normal People with Memory Complaints

Having said all this, there is still a significant population of "the worried well," consisting of people in later middle age and older who are, in fact, perfectly normal cognitively but have concerns about their memory. Studies of this group of people, who are frequently seen in memory disorder clinics, indicate that they are more likely to have mood disorders than AD. Most people in their 50s who have memory complaints fit into this category. Whether such minor mood disturbances predispose to developing AD in a manner similar to the more severe depression symptoms evaluated in the MIRAGE study is not certain. The first author's personal strategy of working with these patients is to listen to them carefully, perform a set of bedside cognitive tests, and assuming that they do well, send them away with reassurances that at this point everything seems fine. An antidepressant or psychiatric evaluation may be suggested if the depressive symptoms are severe enough, and a recommendation may be given to come back for a reevaluation in 6 months to a year if they still feel they have a problem or if their condition gets worse.

MEASURING DEPRESSION

As mentioned previously, depression is typically diagnosed through a clinical interview based upon patient and, sometimes, family member accounts. There is also a tool that may help neurologists notice depressive symptoms in elderly and/or dementia patients. The Cornell Scale for Depression in Dementia is completed by the physician after interviewing both the patient and the caregiver. It has nineteen items that rate mood, behavioral disturbance (such as agitation or slowing), physical signs (such as appetite changes), cyclic functions (such as sleep changes), and ideational disturbances (such as self-esteem problems or thoughts of suicide) on a 0 to 2 scale. All observations are based on the previous week. A total score of 8 or higher may indicate depression.

A second tool used in the doctor's office, the Neuropsychiatric Inventory (NPI), assesses depression as well as other neuropsychiatric symptoms, such as delusions and hallucinations (see next section). The long form of the NPI consists of a structured interview conducted with the caregiver. The short version is a questionnaire completed by the caregiver. Both forms have twelve symptom categories and include ratings on the severity of the symptom and how much it bothers the caregiver. The NPI is an excellent checklist of behaviors that may pose a challenge in AD patients, and it reminds the caregiver to report changes in these areas to the physician.

OTHER NEUROBEHAVIORAL SYMPTOMS

Neurobehavioral symptoms other than depression may be experienced in the moderate stage of AD, but they often disappear as the patient's dementia becomes more severe. Delusions and hallucinations are two common symptoms in moderate AD that are rarely present in MCI. Delusions are false beliefs that are not shared by an individual's culture, but are held with extraordinary certainty and unshakeable conviction, even in the face of contradictory evidence. In AD patients, a common delusion is that a personal item has been stolen. They may even accuse family members of being the perpetrators. It is important to understand that these accusations are part of the disease process. Also, caregivers should not try to argue with the patient because, by definition, delusions are irrational and cannot be swayed with logical argument. The best strategy is redirection, that is, to divert their attention toward something else.

One specific type of delusion, the *Capgras syndrome*, may be especially disturbing to caregivers. In this delusion, the patient believes that the caregiver or other family member is an imposter. The patient acknowledges that the person may look the same, dress the same, and act the same, but nonetheless insist that it is not really the family member. The patient may even become hostile towards the suspected imposter. There is also an object variant of the Capgras syndrome where a person believes an object is not really that object. For example, they may insist that their house really belongs to somebody else, but just happens to appear identical to their own house. A related condition, the *delusional misidentification syndrome*, occurs when the patient misidentifies relatives; for example, confusing his wife with his sister. Incidentally, it is not uncommon for an AD patient to misidentify relatives, especially ones that are not seen frequently. This is only delusional if they refuse to change their opinion when told otherwise. The Capgras syndrome is to be distinguished from simply not recognizing family members at all, which happens late in the course of the disease.

Hallucinations are also quite common in the moderate stage of AD. Hallucinations are a sensory perception that has the compelling sense of reality of a true perception, but they occur without external stimulation of the relevant sensory organ. In other words, a hallucination is seeing, hearing, smelling, tasting, or feeling something that is not there. In AD, hallucinations tend to be visual and are often of deceased relatives, with whom the patient may sometimes seem to be conversing. Ordinarily, the hallucinations of AD are nonthreatening and may not especially disturb the patient, however there are exceptions.

On occasion, hallucinations may turn paranoid. The patient may believe that someone or something is harassing, persecuting, or even threatening her. In rare circumstances, this can lead the patient to actively "defend" herself, possibly causing harm to herself or another person. Effective treatment for delusions and hallucinations may be achieved using the standard AD medications that work on the acetylcholine system, antipsychotic medications, or a combination of the two (see Chapter 9).

Anxiety, manifested by such signs as sighing, being short of breath, and generally being unable to relax, is also witnessed in AD. Separation anxiety may occur when the caregiver has to leave, particularly when the patient is in unfamiliar places. Patients may become agitated, cranky, and resistive when feeling anxious.

Apathy and indifference, unlike the previous three symptoms, are more likely to be seen in the first phase of AD. The patient may change from taking the lead in planning or suggesting activities to being content to be led by the spouse. In addition, hobbies and activities that they used to enjoy may now only be taken up sporadically, if at all. Persistent apathy may be an indication of depression and should be discussed with a physician.

Disinhibition, difficulty in coping with delays, motor disturbances such as pacing, unusual night time behavior, and appetite changes are also commonly documented in AD at various stages. Disinhibition is manifested by acting impulsively, or by such behaviors as talking in a familiar fashion to strangers or saying things that may hurt other people's feelings. Changes in sleep/wake cycles may result in the patient napping frequently during the day, and then becoming active in the middle of the night, disrupting the caregiver's sleep. The tendency of demented patients to become particularly confused and agitated during the evening hours is called "sundowning." This can become prominent during moderate and severe AD stages, and occasionally it can be so severe that a sedating medication is necessary.

Last, perhaps the most problematic behavior in moderate to advanced AD is *wandering*. Patients in the later stages of AD are able to walk around without the benefit of other cognitive skills, because AD generally spares basic motor abilities. They may wander aimlessly and unpredictably. For this reason, nursing homes with specialized Alzheimer's units have locked doors. In general, it is recommended that all AD patients wear a bracelet containing their name, address, phone number, and diagnosis so that they can be easily identified should they become lost. The technology already exists for AD patients to be given a subcutaneous (under the skin) electronic chip implant so that they can be located at any time with the Global Positioning Satellite system. The chip should also contain important medical information, in case the family cannot be immediately located.

Prevalence of Neuropsychiatric Symptoms

The number of potential behavioral disturbances in AD can be daunting for the patient and caregiver alike. Often it is these neuropsychiatric symptoms that are more difficult for the caregiver to cope with than the purely cognitive deficits associated with dementia. Unfortunately, AD patients are highly likely to experience at least one type of problematic

> The number of potential behavioral disturbances in AD can be daunting.

behavior over the course of their illness. The Cardiovascular Health Study discussed previously used the NPI to evaluate other neuropsychiatric symptoms in addition to depression. Overall, almost one-third of MCI and nearly two-thirds of dementia patients had experienced one or more clinically significant neurobehavioral symptoms within the month prior to the survey. Over half of the demented patients had two or more of the twelve symptoms evaluated on the NPI, and 44 percent had three or more. The study also showed that these symptoms generally occurred with similar frequency in patients with other forms of dementia, except for aberrant motor behaviors such as wandering, which were more prevalent in AD patients. Since patients are likely to exhibit one or more neuropsychiatric symptoms, and changes in behavior should be promptly reported to the physician so that possible behavioral and medication treatments can be discussed.

Chapter 9

Medications for Alzheimer's Disease

Chapter Question:
What treatments are available for Alzheimer's disease?

Over the past decade, significant advances have been made in the development of new drugs for Alzheimer's disease, but none provide a cure. Presently, there are three major FDA-approved drugs

> Significant advances have been made in the development of new drugs for Alzheimer's disease, but none provide a cure.

that share a similar mechanism of action: donepezil (Aricept®), rivastigmine (Exelon®), and galantamine (Reminyl®). There is no substantial evidence that one is superior to another. A new drug, memantine (Namenda®) was approved in late 2003 for moderate to severe AD; it has a mechanism of action different from the other drugs. All four AD medications provide some improvement in symptoms and may slow the progression of decline.

DISCLOSURE: THE FIRST STEP TOWARD TREATMENT

FAMILIES ARE SOMETIMES TOLD of the Alzheimer's diagnosis when the patient is absent. This presents a dilemma: Should the family reveal the diagnosis to the patient or should they hide it? Some families feel that informing the patient will cause him to become upset or depressed.

A patient who is not told the diagnosis and the expected course of his illness, however, may not agree to try medication for AD. Understanding his symptoms and being offered medications that may slow the progression of the illness may actually prevent serious depression or apathy by giving the patient a sense of control. In addition, information regarding the stages of AD and the progression of the disease may encourage patients to put legal and financial affairs in order. This will greatly reduce the burden on the caregiver. Consequently, an honest, compassionate disclosure should be considered the first step toward effective management of AD.

The medications that are used in the treatment of AD are summarized in Table 9-1 and discussed in detail in the text that follows.

Table 9-1: Medications Presently Marketed for AD

Medication	Type	Therapeutic Dose	Common Side Effects	Approx Monthly Cost
Donepezil (Aricept®)	Cholinesterase inhibitor	5-10 mg once daily	Nausea, vomiting, diarrhea, leg cramps	$130
Rivastigmine (Exelon®)	Cholinesterase inhibitor	3-6 mg twice daily	Same as donepezil	$150
Galantamine (Reminyl®)	Cholinesterase inhibitor	8-12 mg twice daily	Same as donepezil	$140
Memantine (Namenda®)	Glutamate antagonist	10 mg twice daily	Sedation, constipation	$130

ACETYLCHOLINESTERASE INHIBITORS

In the mid-1970s, scientists discovered evidence suggesting that acetylcholine levels, along with the levels of several other neurotransmitters, were greatly reduced in the brains of AD patients. Acetylcholine is an important neurotransmitter for memory function in the brain. Thus, low levels of this chemical in the brain help explain the memory problems associated with AD.

Early treatment efforts focused on raising acetylcholine levels in the brain by having patients take dietary supplements of lecithin. Lecithin breaks down in the body to form choline, a building block for acetylcholine. Long-term studies of lecithin supplements in AD patients showed that the compound had minimal or no effect on the illness. The results of these studies inspired scientists to pursue a different strategy. Instead of trying to make more acetylcholine, they attempted to prevent it from being broken down (a normal process performed almost continuously). The main enzyme in the body that breaks down acetylcholine into an acetyl group plus a choline group is called *acetylcholinesterase*. The first four drugs on the market share a common mechanism of action: They inhibit acetylcholinesterase. This prevents the breakdown of acetylcholine, making more available for the brain to use.

Cognex®

The first drug available to treat AD by inhibiting acctylcholinesterase was tacrine (Cognex®). It was approved by the Federal Drug Administration (FDA) in 1993. Cognex® was a real breakthrough, but very difficult to use. First, it had to be taken four times a day, which was taxing on the patient and the caregiver. Second, it had a lot of side

> The first drug available to treat AD by inhibiting acetylcholinesterase was tacrine (Cognex®).

effects, especially nausea, vomiting, and diarrhea. Consequently, the dose had to be increased very gradually, and many patients could not tolerate an effective dose of the drug. Third, it frequently caused liver dysfunction, and patients had to have liver blood tests done every other week. Despite these problems, for the first time doctors had at least a partially effective medication to offer patients with AD. The following story tells of the dramatic improvement achieved by a patient of Dr. Dash when Cognex® was introduced:

The patient was a lady in her late 70s who had emigrated from Russia, but her English was reasonably fluent. She lived with her daughter, who brought her in because of declining memory over several years. She was rather quiet and withdrawn, and her initial MMSE score was only 4, indicating severe dementia. I started her on Cognex® at 10 mg four times daily. When I saw her again 6 weeks later, she was a bit better, and her MMSE score had gone up to 8. The dose was increased to 20 mg four times a day, and 6 weeks later her MMSE score had improved to 13. The score jumped to 20 at the 30 mg dose, and, finally, at the maximum dose of 40 mg four times a day, she achieved a score of 26, almost normal! She went from being almost completely dependent on her daughter for the activities of daily living to nearly complete independence—she would even fix meals for her daughter sometimes! This remarkable improvement was maintained for the 2 years that I followed her case.

Aricept®

In 1996, donepezil (Aricept®) was released. This drug proved to be a significant improvement over Cognex®, virtually halting new Cognex® prescriptions. Aricept® is taken only once per day; its side effects are much milder than those of Cognex®; and it has no liver toxicity.

> Aricept® is taken only once per day; its side effects are much milder than those of Cognex®.

Aricept® comes in two doses, 5 and 10 mg, and both are clinically effective. It can be taken with or without food. Typically a patient starts on the 5 mg dose, and after a few weeks the 10 mg dose is tried if there is no problem with tolerance. In general, Aricept® is well tolerated. Mild nausea and diarrhea can be a problem, but they are usually temporary side effects. A very rare side effect is *syncope* (fainting), which can occur with an overdose of the drug. A more common side effect is nightmares. Although the instructions from the manufacturer recommend taking

Aricept® in the evening—because in the clinical studies that was when the medication was given—nightmares can often be avoided simply by taking the medication in the morning. Here is an anecdotal account of a patient who had good improvement with Aricept®:

> *Mr. C was in his mid 70s and was brought in by his wife for an evaluation of declining memory. His initial MMSE score was 18, but after being placed on Aricept® he returned 6 weeks later clearly improved, with an MMSE score of 26. Take a look at his before and after clock drawings in Figure 9-1.*

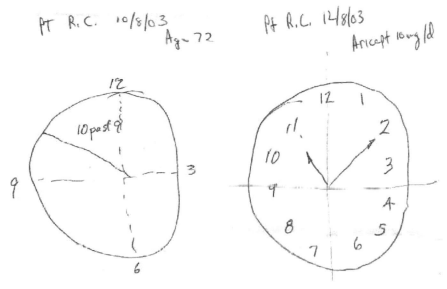

FIGURE 9-1

Clock draw before and after treatment with Aricept®. Patient was told in both cases to set the hands at ten past eleven.

Exelon®

Rivastigmine (Exelon®) was approved by the FDA in 2000. Exelon® inhibits brain acetylcholinesterase, but unlike Aricept®, it also inhibits

Rivastigmine (Exelon®) was approved by the FDA in 2000.

butyrylcholinesterase, another enzyme that breaks down acetylcholine in the liver. In healthy adults, butyrylcholinesterase is found in low levels in the brain. In AD patients, however, more and more of it is found in the brain as the disease progresses, especially in association with amyloid plaques. There is some speculation that this enzyme may be involved in "plaque maturation," which may make the plaque more capable of causing disease. Thus, the theoretical advantage of Exelon® is that it inhibits both types of cholinesterase enzymes, and perhaps interferes with the hypothesized acceleration of the disease process.

The dosage of Exelon® must be increased very slowly. Patients start with 1.5 mg twice a day for at least a month, then increase to 3 mg twice a day. The therapeutic dose is between 3 and 6 mg twice daily. In general, the side effects make it difficult for some people to attain the higher dosage. Exelon® may cause nausea, vomiting, and diarrhea. These problems can be helped by taking the medication with a full meal, increasing the dosage slowly, and, if necessary, using a nonprescription or prescription *antiemetic* (for nausea) and/or an antidiarrheal compound. Symptoms usually improve after a few days. Exelon® must be restarted at the lowest dose and then gradually increased if it has been taken at a therapeutic dose and stopped for more than a week. Resuming the higher dose suddenly may result in severe vomiting. The following story details a patient's progress on Exelon®:

> *An 89-year-old lady came in complaining of progressively worsening memory problems, which her family had also noticed. Two of her older siblings had been diagnosed with AD, and it was clear that she was following in their footsteps. Her MMSE score was 27, which is normal, although she lost all three points on the 3-word recall. Her Q & E score was 5, with 4 points off for recalling only one of the three paired items and 1 point off for naming only twelve animals in a minute's time. As we discussed in Chapter 4, a Q & E score at this level is indicative of mild dementia. Her MRI scan showed atrophy. She started taking Exelon®, and when she returned 2 months later on 3 mg twice daily, both she and her husband were much happier. They both felt her memory had improved. On examination, her MMSE score was still 27, this time with 1 point off for memory and 2 points off on miscellaneous items, but her Q & E score had improved to 1, which is within the normal range.*

Reminyl®

Galantamine (Reminyl®) was approved by the FDA in 2001. It is derived from daffodils, which in herbal folklore were used as a memory potion. Reminyl inhibits brain acetylcholinesterase, but not butyrylcholinesterase.

> Galantamine (Reminyl®) was approved by the FDA in 2001.

The design of Reminyl® improved upon early cholinesterase inhibitors by adding a component that stimulates the release of more acetylcholine. It does this via stimulation of a special receptor for acetylcholine called the *nicotinic receptor*. The additional action of releasing more acetylcholine is nonspecific—meaning the release of other neurotransmitters may also be increased by stimulating the nicotinic receptor.

Reminyl® is taken twice a day, although a once-daily preparation may become available. The starting dose is 4 mg twice per day, which is increased to 8 mg twice per day after 1 month. This dose is therapeutic, but for patients with more advanced AD, it can be increased to 12 mg twice daily. Reminyl® is tolerated somewhat better than Exelon®, but not quite as well as Aricept®. It has the same potential side effects of nausea and diarrhea and, similar to Exelon®, it should be taken with food. The following is an account of one patient's success with Reminyl®:

A 78-year-old African-American man was referred for complaints of hand numbness. This was a simple case of carpal tunnel syndrome (pinched nerve in the wrist). He answered "yes," however, when he was asked if he had noticed any memory problems. He did not seem demented in casual conversation and during the taking of his history, but surprisingly his MMSE score was only 16 with a Q & E score of 6. His MRI showed atrophy, and he was started on Reminyl®. When he returned 3 months later, he brought his wife along, who confirmed that there had been noticeable memory problems, but that they were improving. On 8 mg twice daily, his MMSE score had gone up to 23 and his Q & E score had improved to 3. By the way, his hand was much better after carpal tunnel surgery!

Effectiveness of the Cholinesterase Inhibitors

Drugs must be shown to be effective in order to get FDA approval. To do so, anecdotes such as the ones above are not sufficient. The drugs approved for AD went through similar types of rigorous experiments called "randomized double-blinded placebo controlled trials." AD patients were randomly assigned to either a group receiving the active drug or a group receiving the *placebo* (an inactive pill designed to look the same as the drug pill). Neither the patient nor the doctor knew who received which type of pill, active or placebo (that information was tracked by the company doing the trial). Over the course of the studies, which lasted months, patients were administered various tests of cognitive ability.

The outcome measures included the ADAS-cog (Alzheimer's Disease Association Diagnostic Cognition test), discussed in Chapter 4, and the Clinician's Interview-Based Impression of Change (CIBIC+; plus sign refers to caregiver input). The CIBIC+ surveys the doctor as to his overall impression of the patient (better, worse, same) throughout the study. The doctor answers these questions based upon his interviews with the patient, and he considers the caregiver's impressions as well. The FDA mandates this test because it does not want to approve an AD drug simply because it may produce an improvement of a few points on a neuropsychologic test. They expect the drug to produce a change that is noticeable to another person.

All three of the newer cholinesterase drugs produced a similar pattern. The drug and placebo groups started out with similar test scores. By the twelfth week, an overall improvement was noted in the drug group, as compared to the placebo group, on all measures. The placebo group gradually declined over time, but eventually so did the drug groups. The same pattern persisted whether the drug group consisted of relatively mild AD patients or those in the moderate to severe stages. The degree of maximal improvement was similar among the different drug trials. For example, the ADAS-cog score improved an average of two points on a 70-point scale.

Some drug trials have also included measures of the neurobehavioral symptoms discussed in Chapter 8, such as depression, delusions, and hallucinations. The cholinesterase inhibitor drugs do have an effect on some of these symptoms. In fact, some dementia experts recommend that they be tried first instead of the traditional antidepressant or antipsychotic drugs.

When the effectiveness and tolerability of the three newer cholinesterase inhibitors have been compared to one another, results have been inconclusive. In a 12-week study, Aricept® was better tolerated than Exelon®, but there was no difference in effectiveness. In a 1-year study of Aricept® versus Reminyl®, there was no difference in the main outcome measures although a slight difference of questionable significance in favor of Reminyl® was noted in some of the other measures. A current question of interest is whether one drug might be better than another at different stages of AD. For example, one could logically ask if Exelon® might be better for the later stages of the disease, because it is the only drug that inhibits levels of butyrylcholinesterase, which tends to increase later in the course of the disease.

Realistic Expectations from AD Drug Treatment

Although some patients show clear improvement on the AD drugs, others seem to experience no benefit. But it is important to understand that in AD "no progress is progress." AD invariably progresses over time, and a medication that keeps the status quo is, in fact, therapeutic. If a patient is put on treatment and the family comes back in a few months and says, "Doctor, this medicine is no good; she's not any different," they can be reminded that without treatment she would have likely gotten worse. They can also be reminded that eventually all patients with AD worsen, because none of the available drugs can permanently halt the course of the disease. This does not mean that the drugs do not provide any benefit, because the decline might have been even faster without treatment.

When Should the Patient Start Taking AD Drugs?

Cholinesterase inhibitor drug treatment is recommended for consideration for all patients with AD, and they should begin AD medication as soon as possible after they have received their diagnosis. There is no evidence that patients will build up immunity if medication is started too soon. As discussed below, there is some evidence that the medications work best when started earlier, rather than later. Although early treatment is recommended, it is a point of debate as to whether AD medication should be prescribed to patients with mild cognitive impairment (MCI). (Future research studies are expected to address this issue. Preliminary results of one major trial of the use of Aricept® in MCI will be discussed in Chapter 16.)

On the other end of the spectrum, there is evidence that the cholinesterase inhibitor drugs also work in the moderate to severe stages, although they are FDA-approved only for the mild to moderate stages. Thus, these medications can probably be started up until the terminal stage is reached.

When Should Medications Be Changed?

It can be difficult to tell if a cholinesterase inhibitor is actually helping an individual patient, and so the question often arises as to whether trying one of the alternate medications may be appropriate. The two issues to consider when deciding whether to change medications are *effectiveness* and *tolerability*.

A 6-month trial is recommended when trying an AD medication, unless side effects prevent the patient from continuing to take it. In one study, 70 percent of patients who initially showed no benefit from Aricept® after 3 months eventually showed benefit at 6 months, as com-

> A 6-month trial is recommended when trying an AD medication.

pared to placebo. If there is no indication that the drug is helping, however, and the patient seems to be declining at the same rate as before— or as expected for untreated AD patients (2 to 4 points or more decline in MMSE score per year)—changing medications is a reasonable strategy.

If the drug appears to lose effectiveness over the course of the illness, an alternative strategy is to try increasing the dosage of the medication beyond the recommended limit. In all cases, expectations of what constitutes lack of effectiveness of a drug should be reviewed with a physician.

With respect to tolerability, it is important to accurately attribute the symptoms to the medication. Certain side effects may be caused by the medication, but many can also occur for a variety of other reasons, especially in the elderly. Various strategies, such as taking the medication with food, starting with only half of a pill and increasing very slowly, or temporarily using a medication to help overcome the most common side effects (nausea or diarrhea), are often helpful in getting the patient "over the hump" of staying on the medication. A new strategy option is to try adding Namenda®, because its side effect of constipation may counteract the tendency to diarrhea caused by the cholinesterase inhibitors. Theoretically, Namenda® also has some antinausea properties.

Few studies have been published on the benefits of changing medications, and those that have been published suffer from significant flaws in study design. More research on this topic is needed. It is likely that patients will show individual differences in response to the different drugs. Dr. Clive Ballard has shown, for example, that AD patients respond differently to Exelon® depending on the type of butyryl-cholinesterase gene they possess.

When Should Medication Be Stopped?

A frequently asked question is how long medication should be continued. Although, as mentioned above, there is evidence that drugs continue to help even during the severe stage of the disease, once the patient reaches the terminal phase there is little likelihood of benefit. For example, when the patient is no longer able to walk, has little or no language ability, does not recognize family members, and is reliant on others for virtually all self-care abilities, there is probably little point in continuing to take medication.

A common misconception is that the medications have a time limit as to their effectiveness and, therefore, that there is no point in continuing them after a period of 6 months to a year or so. This comes from studies showing that after an initial increase or stabilization in cognition, patients eventually decline, crossing their starting point during that time period. The fallacy here is that discontinuing the drug will likely result in a sudden drop in cognition, to the point that patients would have reached without treatment in the first place.

In the drug trials with Aricept®, patients were followed after approximately a 6-month treatment period during "washout" times of 3 or 6 weeks in separate studies, during which time they received no medication. A decline was apparent during the 3-week washout, although the treatment groups did not get quite to the level of the placebo group. By 6 weeks, however, patients in the drug groups scored the same as patients in the placebo group: All apparent benefit of the drug had been lost.

Do Cholinesterase Inhibitors Change the Course of AD?

There is some evidence that cholinesterase inhibitors actually modify the course of AD. After the initial drug trials, in which drug groups were compared to placebo groups, patients in the placebo groups were offered the same AD medication as the drug groups. Overall, these patients improved, but in studies of all three drugs, the placebo group did not "catch up" to the performance of the initial drug group. They derived less benefit from the drugs because of the 6-month delay.

Results have been similar in longer studies. One investigation using Reminyl® found that, even after 2 years on the medication, the placebo group that was treated later still scored lower than the initial drug group. Another study with Reminyl® reported a slower rate of decline in AD patients using this drug for 3 years compared to a historical group of untreated controls. A 5-year investigation of Exelon® revealed that, over the course of the study, AD patients declined an average of 6 total points on the MMSE, as compared with an expected decline of 2 to 4 points per year. Last, an anatomic brain comparison of untreated AD patients to those with over 6 months of treatment with Aricept® showed less shrinkage in the hippocampus (see Chapter 3). The slower rate of cognitive decline and hippocampal shrinkage in the treated groups provides evidence that the drugs modify the disease course.

The positive effects on patients using AD drugs bring additional relief to the caregiver and they have the added benefit of possibly saving the family money in the long term. The cost for an AD drug is approximately $130 per month, but cost effectiveness studies have shown that investments in the medication result in savings over the course of the illness because the patient can stay home longer. At least one study has shown that patients treated with Aricept® were able to postpone nursing home placement for an average of almost 2 years longer than untreated patients.

Overall, the studies provide support for the following two extremely important conclusions:

1. Once treatment is started, do not stop.
2. The earlier treatment is started, the better.

Cholinesterase Inhibitors in Non-AD Dementias

Although the cholinesterase inhibitors are FDA-approved only for AD, there is some evidence that they may be effective in treating non-AD dementias. In several studies, both Exelon® and Aricept® have been shown to improve symptoms in dementia with Lewy bodies. Aricept® and Reminyl® have proved promising for treatment of vascular dementia. The cholinesterase inhibitors may also be partially effective in dementias associated with neurologic illnesses, such as multiple sclerosis and Parkinson's disease, and to a limited extent in patients with head trauma. On the other hand, studies with Aricept® have shown no benefit for patients with frontotemporal dementia or the dementia associated with a rare neurologic disease called progressive supranuclear palsy.

MEMANTINE (NAMENDA®): A NEW APPROACH

In late 2003, the FDA approved *memantine* (Namenda®), the newest AD drug released in the United States. Namenda® works on a neurotransmitter system different from the cholinesterase inhibitors; it modifies the

> Namenda® works on a neurotransmitter
> system different from the cholinesterase
> inhibitors; it modifies the glutamate system.

glutamate system. Glutamate is an important neurotransmitter for learning and memory, but excessive amounts can be toxic to cells. Glutamate toxicity may be partly responsible for neuronal death in AD. Namenda® blocks a key glutamate receptor, thereby preventing glutamate toxicity, while still allowing enough glutamate activity to permit normal learning and memory function in most people.

Namenda® has few side effects in most patients, no evidence of safety problems has surfaced, and there are no significant interactions with other medications. The recommended dosage is 10 mg twice a day. The drug is approved only for moderate to severe AD. In drug trials, these more advanced AD patients showed stabilization on most measures, whereas the placebo groups declined. The initial trial of Namenda® in mild AD patients was not successful. In 2004, however, a larger study of mild to moderate patients proved promising. Hence, Forest Labs, the company that markets Namenda® in the United States, is pursuing FDA approval for the use of the drug with mild-stage AD patients.

One study compared the efficacy of prescribing Namenda® for moderate AD patients already taking Aricept® to continuing treatment with Aricept® alone. The combination group did better overall than the Aricept®-only group. Combination trials of Namenda® with all three major cholinesterase inhibitor drugs are in progress, as well as trials comparing the drugs in a *monotherapy* design (one drug per patient group).

NON-DRUG TREATMENTS FOR AD PATIENTS

Various behavioral strategies have been proposed for trying to preserve and improve cognition in AD. Unfortunately, the few studies available have not been encouraging. E. Farina conducted a study that compared two training strategies in mild to moderate AD patients. The first strategy involved an attempt to capitalize on a relatively preserved memory type: procedural memory. Patients performed various activities of daily living—such as setting a table, identifying currency, and opening and closing a door lock in a repetitious fashion—during twice daily 45-minute sessions for 5 weeks under the supervision of a physical therapist. The second strategy was based on the use of residual cognitive functions, and required patients to perform various memory, language, and visuospatial tasks, such as recalling numbers, naming pictures, and working through mazes. Both groups improved on a measure of functional skills sensitive to mild changes after the training sessions, but no difference was observed in the activities of daily living scales that measure larger changes. In addition, after 3 months, both groups had returned to baseline performance—meaning there was no lasting benefit from the training.

In a similar study led by Cahn-Weiner, patients with mild AD participated in a memory training program. Compared to a no-training patient group, the trained group could better recall the items presented during the testing sessions. Unfortunately, there were no differences between the groups in their ability to recall newly presented information. In other words, like the patients in Farina's study, the trained patients could not apply their new skills to learning new information.

Although the results of specific cognitive training programs have been disappointing, environmental risk factors are important in AD. For example, there is evidence that staying mentally active can help *prevent* the development of AD. In addition, it is recommended that people with AD be encouraged to continue their regular hobbies as long as possible. Perhaps in the future, cognitive training combined with the right AD medications will be able to enhance new learning.

DOCTORS NEED HELP, TOO

Statistics indicate that doctors could do a better job of diagnosing and treating AD. As of 2000, there were an estimated 1,200,000 Americans with mild AD, less than half of whom had been diagnosed. Of those who had been diagnosed, approximately one-fourth were not being actively treated. Even among patients with moderate AD, only half of the estimated 1,000,000 had been diagnosed, and, again, one-fourth of them were not being treated. Of the 300,000 people in the severe AD stage, the vast majority had been diagnosed, but about three-fourths were not being treated.

Doctors need more education in the diagnosis and treatment of AD. Many are not familiar with the available treatment options because the suggested treatments are fairly new. By becoming an informed patient

> Doctors need more education in the diagnosis and treatment of AD.

or caregiver, effective treatment options can be realized. Search for a knowledgeable physician, discuss early drug intervention, and continue to explore newly released FDA-approved treatments.

Chapter 10

Treatments for Behavioral Symptoms and Other Complications of Alzheimer's

Chapter Question:
Mom's hallucinating—can medication help?

Chapter 10 reviews the medications and behavioral strategies available for treating the depression, psychotic symptoms, and sleep disturbances that can complicate Alzheimer's disease. In addition, treatment for AD-related seizures is discussed as well as delirium, a condition that may occur shortly after hospitalization. The majority of the medications discussed in this chapter are summarized in Table 10-1.

TREATMENT FOR DEPRESSION

A VARIETY OF BEHAVIORAL PROBLEMS can complicate the course of AD, most often in the moderate or severe stages of the disease. These behaviors can be emotionally taxing on the patient and family. Successful treatment should provide considerable relief, especially to the primary caregiver. Depression is one of the more common problems

> Behavioral problems can complicate the course of AD.

107

Table 10-1: Medications for Behavioral Symptoms

Symptom	Type of Medicine	Names
Depression	SSRI	Prozac®, Zoloft®, Lexapro® Paxil®, others
Hallucinations, delusions	Atypical antipsychotic	Risperdal®, Geodon®, Abilify®, Seroquel®, Zyprexa
Insomnia	Benzodiazepine-related	Ambien®, Sonata®
Restless legs syndrome	Dopamine agonist	Mirapex®, Requip®
Aggression	Atypical antipsychotic	See above
	Anticonvulsants	Lamictal®, Depakote®
Anxiety, agitation	Benzodiazepine-related	Ativan®, Xanax®
Hypersexuality	Hormone	Provera®

experienced with many progressive illnesses. Depression has a complicated relationship with AD. As discussed in Chapter 8, depression can be confused with AD, result from AD, and can even be a risk-factor for the development of AD.

Pharmacologic (drug) therapy for depression commonly includes tricyclic antidepressants or selective serotonin reuptake inhibitors. Tricyclic antidepressants, such as amitriptyline (Elavil®), should be avoided with AD because they have an anticholinergic action that may exacerbate cognitive symptoms. Selective serotonin reuptake inhibitors (SSRIs) can be used by AD patients. Some theories on the causes of depression suggest that low levels of serotonin contribute to depressed symptoms. SSRIs can increase the amount of serotonin available in the brain, and they are relatively free from side effects. SSRIs include the popular drugs fluoxetine (Prozac®), paroxetine (Paxil®), sertraline (Zoloft®), and escitalopram (Lexapro®).

Although, in general, the SSRIs have been extensively studied in depression, only a few studies have investigated their effectiveness in treating the depression associated with AD. Several studies using Zoloft® and Prozac® with AD patients revealed conflicting results, although generally speaking they tended to be beneficial. Part of the reason for the inconclusive results is due to the assumption that the same causes used to explain depression in otherwise healthy adults are the same causes in AD. Progressive dementia affects all the neurotransmitter systems, and boosting serotonin levels may not be enough for all depressed AD patients. A trial of SSRI medication in a depressed AD patient is certainly warranted, however, and may result in symptom relief.

There are also nonpharmacologic strategies that can help when used alone or with medication. Caregivers and patients should focus on two main goals, especially if the depression seems linked to the diagnosis of AD or frustration because of the loss of function. The first goal should be to try to accept the diagnosis and prognosis of Alzheimer's disease. Education and familial support can improve a person's ability to cope with loss. In addition, support groups consisting of AD patients or patients and caregivers can provide a comfortable forum where the patient and family can express their fears, sadness, and anger.

A second goal should be to improve the patient's quality of life. The patient should be encouraged to engage in activities that he has always enjoyed, develop new interests that he can perform despite some loss of function, and participate as much as possible in household and medical decisions. A sense of control, independence, and being needed can improve a person's perspective and add purpose to their lives. These aspects of life are important in order for everyone to feel happy and secure, but they may be especially difficult to achieve for someone who is diagnosed with a progressive illness.

TREATMENT OF PSYCHOTIC SYMPTOMS

There is limited evidence that the cholinesterase inhibitors are helpful in the treatment of psychotic symptoms in AD, including hallucinations (seeing or hearing things that are not there) and delusions (fixed, false beliefs). For example, in a study with Exelon® in moderate dementia, over 60 percent of the patients with hallucinations improved with drug treatment, compared with only 20 percent on placebo. If the patient is already using a cholinesterase inhibitor, however, and begins experiencing psychotic symptoms, an antipsychotic may be useful.

The older antipsychotic medications worked primarily by blocking the receptor for the neurotransmitter dopamine. Excessive dopamine has been linked to schizophrenia, a disease in which hallucinations and delusions are common. Unfortunately, these drugs, such as haloperidol (Haldol®), can have severe adverse reactions in dementia patients, especially those with Lewy body dementia, which is often confused with AD. Elderly patients are generally more prone to developing side effects from the older antipsychotic drugs, including muscle rigidity and *tardive dyskinesia*, a movement disorder in which constant movements of the mouth and tongue develop, and which may persist permanently even when the drug is stopped.

The newer antipsychotic medications also block dopamine receptors, but in addition they affect other neurotransmitter systems. In fact, there is some evidence that shows they increase the levels of acetylcholine. This makes them a better choice for AD patients. Some examples include quetiapine (Seroquel®), olanzapine (Zyprexa®), risperidone (Risperdal®), aripiprazole (Abilify®), and ziprasidone (Geodon®). All of these drugs have different side effect profiles that can sometimes be used to advantage. For example, Seroquel® is particularly sedating, so it is especially useful in patients who are very agitated. Limited studies on Risperdal® and Zyprexa® have shown efficacy in treating the psychotic symptoms associated with AD. Unfortunately, the authors are unaware of any studies that have carefully evaluated the changes in cognition associated with the new antipsychotics. CATIE—Clinical Antipsychotic Trials of Intervention Effectiveness—is a large study that is investigating this question. One caution about these new medicines is that they have been associated with elevated blood sugar levels and diabetes and, hence, monitoring of glucose levels is recommended.

To help alleviate symptoms that do arise, family members should not argue with patients about their delusional symptoms. By definition, delusions are irrational beliefs, and, thus, logical discussion will not sway them. Caregivers and family members should be sympathetic, but do not endorse the hallucinations. For example, ask patients if they feel afraid, but state that you do not see or hear what they are talking about. Reassure them that they are safe, and try to distract them with another activity. Sometimes the "hallucination" is actually an illusion. In other words, they only misperceive an object or noise in the environment. In this case, it can be helpful to simply identify the object.

COMMON SLEEP DISORDERS AND TREATMENT

Sleep complaints are common among elderly people, but can be especially problematic in AD patients. Unfortunately, very few scientific studies have been done to evaluate the use of sleep medications in dementia, and virtually no studies have evaluated the effectiveness of nonpharmacologic maneuvers, such as sleep hygiene. There are three

> Sleep complaints are common among elderly people, but can be especially problematic in AD patients.

types of sleep problems, all of which can be interrelated: sleeping too much during the day, not being able to go to sleep at night, and difficulty staying asleep.

Frequent naps during the day in dementia patients could be a symptom of their illness; for example, dementia with Lewy bodies. It is important to be sure that the person does not suffer from a sleep disorder. Sleep disorders typically develop in midlife or even earlier, it is not uncommon for them to go undiagnosed for years. Proper diagnosis of a sleep disorder requires a *polysomnogram*, which involves monitoring that is done while a person spends the night in a sleep lab.

Sleep Apnea

The most common sleep disorder that causes excessive daytime sleepiness is *sleep apnea*, which is especially prevalent in overweight individuals. Loud snoring at night is characteristic of sleep apnea, along with pauses that may last many seconds, followed by gasping breaths. Sleep is nonrestorative, which results in the person falling asleep easily during the day. In addition, individuals with sleep apnea may become irritable and complain of fatigue.

This condition occurs when the airway passage is blocked by overly relaxed muscles during sleep. When the oxygen level in the blood falls, the brain responds by triggering a brief arousal that causes a person to take a breath. This cycle repeats throughout the night, disrupting the natural ability of sleep to restore brain function. The arousals last only a few seconds, and are often not remembered, although waking up at night does occur. Sleep apnea is also associated with nocturnal urination, which in men may be confused with prostate problems. Sleep disruption can worsen cognition in anyone. If sleep apnea contributes to a decrease in cognitive functioning in a dementia patient, then successful treatment may result in some improvement.

Insomnia

Insomnia affects individuals of all ages, but it is more prevalent in older adults. Symptoms include trouble falling asleep, repeated waking during the night, and early arousals. As a result, people suffering from insomnia may be tired during the day, experience symptoms of sleep deprivation (such as difficulty paying attention), and become irritable. Everyone has trouble falling asleep occasionally. However, persons with chronic insomnia have so much trouble with sleep quality that they become anxious just thinking about falling asleep. This anxiety can also contribute to problems falling asleep and further perpetuate the cycle.

Restless Legs Syndrome

Restless legs syndrome is a sleep disturbance marked by a compulsion to move the legs, typically at rest. Patients report a "creepy-crawly" or itchy sensation that is relieved momentarily by leg movements. These sensations often cause difficulty falling asleep. Once asleep, there may be additional problems with periodic movements. As with sleep apnea, these movements cause micro-arousals resulting in poorer quality sleep and excessive daytime sleepiness.

REM Behavior Disorder

REM behavior disorder is a rare disorder characterized by movement during REM sleep. The person may act out dreams, sometimes violently, and may recall especially vivid dreams. Grunting, shouting, and sleepwalking are also common. REM behavior disorder can precede Lewy body dementia by several years.

Confusion in the Middle of the Night

Dementia patients do not have to suffer from a sleep disorder for there to be problems during the night. They may simply wake up in the middle of the night to go to the bathroom and become disoriented and confused. They may even get dressed, perhaps thinking that they are still working and have to leave shortly. Some of this behavior is relatively harmless, although bothersome for other family members. A more dangerous situation arises when the patient decides to leave the house. The house should be secure to prevent such activity. In addition, a simple night-light may be enough to help orient a person and guide her safely back to bed. Frequent sleep disruptions will inevitably result in daytime napping. Prescription and behavioral remedies should be considered in order to avoid a maladaptive cycle.

Medications for Sleep Problems

Medications for sleep can be a double-edged sword. Some can cause dependency and may worsen confusion in dementia patients. Nonprescription sleeping aids often contain medications with antihistamine or anticholinergic properties, which are generally not recommended for AD patients, although anecdotally some caregivers report success with medications such as Tylenol PM®. The older benzodiazepine drugs, such as Valium®, are also discouraged because they have long-lasting effects. Trazadone®, an older antidepressant with sedating qualities, is commonly used as a sleeping aid, but some patients can have a marked increase in daytime confusion.

113

In the treatment of insomnia, zolpidem (Ambien®) is recommended for people who wake up too early, and zaleplom (Sonata®) is useful for people who have trouble falling but not staying asleep. For REM sleep disorder, clonazepam (Klonopin®) is effective in doses of 0.5 to 2 mg at night. Melatonin, a natural hormone that promotes sleep, is available over the counter. However, a study of melatonin in AD patients with sleep disturbances failed to show any definite benefit. If tried, it should be given at sunset to mimic the natural body pattern of melatonin secretion.

Finally, there is also some evidence that cholinesterase inhibitors can improve symptoms of sleep-wake cycle disturbances. This reinforces the recommendation that all mild to moderate AD patients should be on one of these drugs.

Behavioral Treatment for Sleep Problems

Behavioral changes should be used to help improve sleep over time, because it is generally not recommended that anyone use prescription sleep aids for a long period of time. A popular strategy suggested by physicians is to follow the principles of sleep hygiene. Sleep hygiene, outlined in Table 10-2, is a system of behavioral and environmental changes designed to improve sleep. By adopting these guidelines, sleep habits will most likely be manageable, and prescription drugs will only be necessary occasionally.

Table 10-2: Principles of Sleep Hygiene

1. Make sure the sleeping environment is quiet and restful. Discourage television, as it tends to be arousing. Soft classical music can be helpful.
2. A warm evening bath may help the person to relax.
3. Avoid stimulants, such as caffeine, in the evening.
4. Limit fluids prior to bedtime and make sure the person has used the restroom.
5. If the person wakes too early, try going to bed later.
6. Arouse the person at the same time every morning, regardless of how little sleep they may have had the night before.
7. Encourage exercise during the day, but avoid it in the evening hours.
8. Avoid daytime napping, especially in the early evening.
9. Increase natural light exposure during the day.

Anger and Irritability

Anger and irritability are common in the later stages of dementia, and they can be exacerbated or caused by depression or sleep disturbances. Sleep quality and depression should be evaluated if a person has these symptoms. Anger and irritability can also be a result of discomfort. Language disturbances may prevent the patient from expressing pain or problems with constipation and hunger. Try to speak gently, give

> Anger and irritability are common in the later stages of dementia.

instructions as simply as possible, and use distraction if the person becomes belligerent. It is helpful to remember that these are symptoms of the disease. The behavior is not some willful character flaw. If depression, sleep disturbances, and discomfort have been ruled out, and the anger and irritability persist, then medication may be necessary. Antidepressants (such as Zoloft®), antianxiety drugs (such as Xanax®), or antipsychotics (such as Seroquel®) may be tried.

Aggression and Inappropriate Sexual Behavior

Aggression and inappropriate sexual behavior can surface in the later stages of AD, as the illness affects larger portions of the brain. If a patient

> Aggression and inappropriate sexual behavior can surface in the later stages of AD.

begins having aggressive outbursts, the caregiver may first want to try to determine whether there is a particular trigger. In general, there are several strategies that may reduce the outbursts:

• Rephrase instructions so that they sound less demanding.
• Do not physically attempt to move or redirect the patient.

- Introduction of a pet, the use of soothing music, and pleasant smells (aromatherapy) may help to create a calming atmosphere.
- Restructure the environment so that it is less confusing. For example, increase the lighting, decrease the clutter, and keep the person in the same two or three rooms.
- Obviously, dementia patients should not have access to weapons.

The physician may recommend medication if problems with aggression cannot be managed behaviorally, or if inappropriate sexual behavior has become bothersome. Inderal (Propranolol®) and valproate (Depakote®) have been beneficial in treating some patients for aggression, and medroxyprogesterone (Provera®), a female hormone, may be helpful for both aggression and inappropriate sexual behaviors in men. The atypical antipsychotic agents are usually tried first in these situations, however.

Anxiety, Agitation, and Motor Behaviors

Anxiety, which is often accompanied by restlessness, agitation, and repetitive behaviors, is another common neurobehavioral symptom in AD. It is critical to assess whether some physical condition may be caus-

> Anxiety is another common neurobehavioral symptom in AD.

ing agitation in people with more advanced AD, who are not able to fully express themselves, particularly if the problem has started suddenly. The same physical problems that may result in anger and irritability, such as constipation, pain, or hunger, should be evaluated. If discomfort is not to blame, and the problems escalate or last several weeks, the patient may be offered an antidepressant medication, a sedative, an antianxiety medication, or an anticonvulsant.

If a behavior is especially intense or becomes unmanageable, a short-acting benzodiazepine, such as lorazepam (Ativan®), can help. In general, long-term use of benzodiazepines is not recommended. If it cannot be avoided, then alprazolam (Xanax®) may be considered. Buspirone (BuSpar®) is a nonbenzodiazepine antianxiety medication that can be tried, but it is not nearly as effective as the benzodiazepines. Lastly, treatment with anticonvulsant medications, such as lamotrigine (Lamictal®) or Depakote®, can sometimes alleviate anxiety.

In general, a relatively sudden change in any of the above symptoms may reflect the development of some medical condition (e.g., a urinary tract infection) that is causing the discomfort to the person. A medical evaluation is necessary to exclude such conditions.

Epilepsy and AD

A seizure is a sudden, abnormal electrical discharge that interrupts normal brain function. Epilepsy is defined as repeated, unprovoked seizures. Epilepsy and seizures occur in about 10 percent of AD patients, often not until the moderate or severe stages. There are several different types of seizures. The most severe are *generalized seizures* (in older terminology, grand mal). These are dramatic events where the patient loses consciousness, stiffens, and shakes, usually for a few minutes. Tongue biting and incontinence are common. It may take the patient hours or even a day or two to recover. The more common, and often undetected, type of seizure in AD are *partial complex seizures* (formerly termed petit mal). These seizures are more subtle. A typical event might consist of a sudden change in consciousness, often accompanied by subtle movements of the mouth and face or complex movements in the hands lasting for a few minutes. For example, the patient may have a staring episode, exhibit some chewing and lip-smacking movements of the mouth and seem to fumble with his shirt buttons, during which time he does not respond to questions or commands. These events tend to recur in the same way for a given patient. Sometimes it can be difficult to say if an AD patient is having a partial seizure or is just "off in his own world" and not reacting to the environment for reasons other than seizures. However, the presence of the repetitive motor movements and the time-limited, stereotyped character of partial complex seizures helps to distinguish them from benign behavioral changes that accompany

117

AD. In addition, there are many other possible causes for loss of consciousness, such as irregular heart rhythms, blood sugar levels that are too high or too low and so on.

A first seizure requires immediate medical evaluation, as there are many possible causes. However, if the series of tests, usually including a head CT, EEG, and various blood tests, does not reveal some other cause, the seizure is probably due to an irritative effect on the brain by the Alzheimer pathology itself.

Although a diagnosis of epilepsy requires a minimum of two seizures, most AD patients will be prescribed anticonvulsant medication after the first seizure with the hopes of preventing others. There are numerous medications available for the treatment of seizures, ranging from the older anticonvulsants, like phenytoin (Dilantin®), to the newer drugs, such as zonisamide (Zonegran®), lamotrigine (lamictal), and many others. The more recent medications although more expensive, tend to have fewer side effects and drug interactions. The goal of treatment is to completely eliminate seizures with a minimum of side effects, and fortunately, this is frequently possible in the epilepsy associated with AD.

Usually not seen until the late stages of AD is *myoclonus*. These are isolated, sudden jerking movements, usually of one limb. Myoclonus can be an epileptic phenomenon and may respond to treatment with the right anticonvulsant.

SYMPTOMS ASSOCIATED WITH HOSPITALIZATION

Individuals with AD are at high risk for developing *delirium* when they are hospitalized. Delirium is an acute medical problem that can result from many contributing factors. It is characterized by a fluctuating level of alertness, hallucinations, disorientation, agitation, and inattentiveness. Delirium is a serious cause of illness and death. Being in a hospital can be stressful for anyone, but for an advanced AD patient it can be particularly terrifying. They are in an unfamiliar environment, feel ill, and are subjected to procedures that may be frightening and uncomfortable. Patients may require restraints to prevent them from harming themselves, and they are often given potent sedatives. Unfortunately, even when the cause of the delirium is treated, many advanced AD patients do not fully recover and may seem worse than before.

Sharon Inouye helped pioneer the *Elder Life Program*, which can help reduce the risk and severity of delirium in hospitalized patients. Her recommendations for easing the difficulties of the hospital setting are outlined in Table 10-3. In addition, the family should bring familiar items from home to help keep the person comfortable and oriented. Treatment with a cholinesterase inhibitor should begin or be continued.

Table 10-3: Delirium Prevention Measures

1. Have an orientation board with the names of the care team members and the day's schedule visible. Review with the patient.
2. Communicate frequently to reorient the patient to date and location.
3. Perform a relaxation protocol at bedtime: warm drink, relaxation tape or music, and back massage.
4. Reschedule medications and procedures to allow sleep.
5. Try to have the patient move as much as possible using range of motion exercises. A physical therapist can be helpful in this regard.
6. For the hearing impaired, make sure hearing aids are available.
7. Have visual aids available for those with visual impairment (such as glasses, fluorescent tape on call bell, and telephone with illuminated keypad).
8. Make sure the patient is drinking enough; dehydration can aggravate delirium.

CONCLUDING REMARKS

A variety of complicating symptoms can occur over the course of the illness in Alzheimer's patients. Simple explanations, as well as the more complex medical causes, should be evaluated in each case. Behavioral treatments are free from side effects and involve lifestyle changes that can improve symptoms. When medication is necessary, remember to avoid drugs that can cause confusion and decrease cognitive function. Successful treatment of these co-occurring problems can improve the quality of life and functioning of the person with AD.

Chapter 11

Alternative Treatments for Alzheimer's

Chapter Question:
Can vitamins and herbs help?

This chapter reviews the use of several vitamins, herbs, hormones, and other medications in the treatment of AD. Most of the studies so far regarding these agents are either inconclusive or show no benefit, but some do merit further investigation.

ANTIOXIDANTS

A s ALZHEIMER'S DISEASE PROGRESSES, it attacks different brain areas. Inflammation is one natural response by the body's defense systems to this and other disease processes. Inflammatory cells can be activated when there is a wound, such as cut on the finger, or destruction of tissue because of disease. These cells clean up debris and attack foreign invaders. The chemicals released to accomplish these functions can have toxic side effects, however. In particular, they can trigger a chemical reaction with oxygen (called *oxidation*) that releases free radicals as a byproduct.

Free radicals recruit other molecules in their search for electrical stability and initiate a series of actions that can destroy innocent cells and structures in the process. One of the body's natural control systems for free radicals utilizes antioxidants, such as vitamins E and C. In AD, and even mild cognitive impairment (MCI), there is some evidence that antioxidant levels are reduced. How this association is related to the disease process is still unknown, as is whether or not antioxidants can help in the treatment of AD. Studies are investigating these questions.

Vitamin E

An important role of antioxidants is to bind to free radicals in order to stabilize and thus neutralize them. Vitamin E is a vitamin obtained by eating fruits and vegetables; its main job is to serve as an antioxidant. A research team, lead by Mary Sano, investigated the effectiveness of large doses of vitamin E supplements in the treatment of AD. Patients in the vitamin group took 1000 IU (international units) of vitamin E each day. The recommended daily allowance is only 30 IU. After two years, more patients in the placebo group had died or severely deteriorated in comparison to the vitamin E group.

Unfortunately, as of this writing, the Sano team is the only group to have addressed this question and the results, although promising, should be replicated to be considered valid. Still, the study was provocative enough for the American Academy of Neurologists to recommend that AD patients take vitamin E at the dosage of 1,000 IU twice a day. This dose is generally well tolerated; however, some people have trouble with easy bruising or diarrhea. At this time there is no information on the possible effectiveness of lower doses of vitamin E.

As this book was going to press, an article appeared that challenged the safety of vitamin E supplements. Dr. E. R. Miller of Johns Hopkins and colleagues performed a meta-analysis of 11 studies done with high dose (400 IU or greater) vitamin E supplements in a variety of diseases. Although most of these studies by themselves showed little change of the risk of death with the supplements, when they were all added together they actually pointed to vitamin E causing a small increase in the risk of death. It is unclear if these results will generalize to healthy people taking vitamin E or if they apply to AD. The Sano study cited above was one of two studies in which vitamin E tended towards producing a lower risk of death. Although the Miller study produced a great deal of media publicity, there are several trials involving vitamin E in MCI and AD that are still in progress that should provide additional information on its safety and efficacy.

Vitamin C

Vitamin C (ascorbic acid) has antioxidant properties similar to vitamin E and helps to neutralize free radicals in the body. There has been no formal evaluation of vitamin C in the treatment of AD. However, there are several studies investigating the effectiveness of vitamins C and E in the prevention or delay of dementia (see Chapter 12).

THE B VITAMINS

High levels of homocysteine have been associated with stroke and dementia. Homocysteine is an amino acid (building block of protein) that is normally converted to other amino acids for use by the cells of the body. When the level of homocysteine gets too high, it can cause cholesterol to change to low-density lipoprotein (LDL), which is more damaging to arteries than high-density lipoprotein (HDL). In addition, high homocysteine levels can cause the blood to clot more easily, increasing the risk of blood vessel blockages. The B vitamins help process homocysteine into the helpful amino acids. Low levels of folic acid, B_6, or B_{12} are associated with high levels of homocysteine (see Chapter 4)

It has been suggested that the B vitamins be used to treat AD, because AD patients can have high homocysteine levels. Several studies addressing this proposal have shown mixed results. Used alone, folic acid and B_{12} do not appear to have a benefit. When combined, however, they may reduce homocysteine levels and, in one study, resulted in an improvement in AD patients who initially had elevated homocysteine levels. Researchers are evaluating the usefulness of the B vitamins in treating AD.

GINGKO BILOBA

The herb gingko biloba has been used for centuries in China and is widely used in Europe for the treatment of AD. Gingko extracts have some antioxidant properties, and there is some evidence that gingko inhibits the formation of β-amyloid, a protein that forms the amyloid plaques seen in the brains of AD patients. Patient trials using gingko have provided little solid evidence for or against its use in AD. In fact, in a review in *Scientific American*, lead author Paul Gold concluded that although there was some evidence in favor of gingko's usefulness in AD, there simply was not enough data to recommend routine use. Fortunately, the National Institute of Health (NIH) is sponsoring a large clinical trial of gingko.

There are some properties that should be considered if gingko is suggested by the patient's physician. In general, gingko is well tolerated, but it does have some potential serious side effects, including a tendency to cause bleeding. A typical dosage is 120 mg daily, divided into two or three doses. As with all herbal preparations, the amounts of the various active ingredients are not standardized.

HUPERZINE A

Huperzine A is a chemical isolated from a Chinese herb, *Huperzia serrata*. It acts as a cholinesterase inhibitor, thus increasing the amount of acetylcholine available for use in the brain. It is used in China for the treatment of AD, and at least one study has shown that it is more effective than placebo, and results in memory, cognitive, and behavioral improvements in AD patients. It is recommended that huperzine A and the standard cholinesterase inhibitors used for the treatment of AD not be used together, because there have been no investigations regarding this combined usage. In addition, patients should try the FDA-approved cholinesterase inhibitors, such as Aricept®, first, because more evidence is available regarding results.

MELISSA OFFICINALIS (LEMON BALM)

Melissa officinalis, also known as *lemon balm*, binds to acetylcholine receptors and may enhance activity of this neurotransmitter. It has a mild sedative or calming effect. The first study using this herb in AD was performed in Iran and published in 2003. This small study revealed that the lemon balm group achieved better test scores after 18 weeks than the placebo group. There were no significant side effects, and the herb-treated group reported less agitation. More investigation will clarify the usefulness of this herb in AD treatment.

HYDERGINE

Hydergine (ergoloid mesylates) is developed from a fungus found on rye. It can help stabilize brain oxygen levels and increase brain neurotransmitter levels. It was approved by the FDA in 1978 for treating "idiopathic decline in mental capacity" (idiopathic means disease related to no known cause), and it is used in many countries for the treatment of dementia. Studies conducted over the last 30 years provide, at best, modest evidence as to its efficacy in treating AD. Hydergine is relatively safe and well tolerated, with a possible therapeutic dose of approximately 6 to 12 mg a day. With the advent of the more thoroughly tested cholinesterase inhibitors for AD treatment, hydergine is not widely used.

CHELATION AND CLIOQUINOL

Several metal ions (particularly copper, zinc, and iron) interact with the β-amyloid proteins in complex ways that tend to enhance toxicity by promoting aggregation. There is limited evidence that suggests AD patients have elevated serum copper levels. Chelation therapy involves a series of treatments aimed at "detoxifying" the body of metal. It has been offered as a cure for almost any disease, including AD. Chelation therapy has not been tested in AD. Clioquinol is an older type of antibiotic that has some chelating properties. Interestingly, results of a study with clioquinol in AD showed some evidence of effectiveness, and larger studies are planned.

ANTIBIOTICS

Traces of a common bacterium, *Chlamydia pneumoniae*, have been noted in the brain autopsies of AD patients. This discovery has lead to a radically different theory of AD involving bacterial infection. Mark Loeb from McMaster University conducted a clinical trial using a combination of two antibiotics, doxycycline and rifampin, to treat AD patients. Preliminary results showed that AD patients who had taken the drugs did better than the patients who took placebo, although they could find no difference before and after treatment in the infection rates with the *Chlamydia* bacterium. It is not recommended that antibiotics be used for the treatment of AD, because research in this area is limited and inconclusive.

NONSTEROIDAL ANTI-INFLAMMATORY AGENTS

Nonsteroidal anti-inflammatory agents (NSAIDs) are the world's most widely used drugs, including nonprescription agents such as aspirin, ibuprofen (Advil® and Motrin®), and naprosyn (Aleve®), and prescription brands such as celecoxib (Celebrex®) and rofecoxib (Vioxx®), although the latter drug has been withdrawn from the market. Several studies have suggested that people who take NSAIDs regularly (for example, those with arthritis) are less likely to develop AD, presumably because of the anti-inflammatory affects of NSAIDs on the brain. Large trials have been com-

> People who take NSAIDs regularly are less likely to develop AD.

pleted with naprosyn, Celebrex®, and Vioxx®, and there were no differences reported in any outcome for patients taking these NSAIDs compared to placebo. During the course of the study, evidence surfaced that showed certain NSAIDs, such as ibuprofen, but not the NSAIDs used in the above studies, interfered with β-amyloid aggregation. Therefore, despite the negative studies on NSAIDs thus far, the question remains as to whether the NSAIDs that interfere with β-amyloid aggregation, which have thus far not been tested, might still be effective.

ESTROGEN

Initial studies of estrogen, a female hormone, looked promising for the treatment of AD. The positive effects noted in animals did not carry over into the human population, however. Short-term trials of estrogen in AD patients failed to show any benefit. Larger, long-term trials showed that, contrary to expectations, women who took estrogen or estrogen/progesterone supplements actually had an increased risk of developing dementia, as well as hypertension, stroke, and heart attack. The only apparent benefit was a lower rate of bone fractures and osteoporosis. Consequently, women are now advised to use estrogen only for short-term control of menopausal symptoms, such as hot flashes, but not as a long-term preventive for other health reasons.

STATINS

Statin drugs, such as lovastatin (Mevacor®), simvistatin (Zocor®), and atorvastatin (Lipitor®), are used to lower cholesterol and, thus, reduce the risk of heart disease. Several studies have shown a significant reduction in the risk of developing AD in people taking statin drugs. High cholesterol levels are, at best, only a modest risk factor for the development of AD. It is hypothesized that the lowered risk in these groups is the result of the effects of the statin drugs on β-secretase and α-secretase activity. To review, β-secretase has a pathologic reaction with amyloid proteins that encourages the aggregation of amyloid plaques, but α-secretase is involved in the normal, healthy breakdown of amyloid proteins. These enzymes reside in the cell membrane, and their activity is affected by the amount of cholesterol that is present there. Statin drugs inhibit β-secretase activity and enhance α-secretase activity by lowering the amount of cholesterol in the cell membrane.

Large-scale investigations into the effectiveness of statin drugs in the treatment of AD are now being conducted. As of the time of this writing, some smaller studies have been completed that show mixed results. Michael Simon and colleagues report that Zocor® resulted in lower cerebrospinal fluid amyloid levels compared to placebo, but there was no significant improvement on cognitive testing. Other studies have failed to find any difference in plasma β-amyloid levels in AD patients treated with Zocor® and Lipitor®. Thus treatment with statins is not yet recommended for Alzheimer's disease, because the statin drugs can have significant side effects, including muscle pain and weakness. They are also expensive, and they may differ significantly with one another regarding possible benefits. Of course, AD patients may still benefit from these drugs when they are prescribed to treat elevated cholesterol levels.

THE TREATMENT "DU JOUR"

It seems as though new treatments for AD are being proposed on a weekly basis. It is important to ask some basic questions, however, before trying any new treatment. First, is the treatment approved by the FDA? If so, it means the drug has gone through rigorous testing for both safety and efficacy. If not, it does not necessarily mean that the drug will not work. Some drugs are out of patent protection, similar to the antibiotics mentioned above, and getting FDA approval is an expensive process. Sometimes, when alternative uses for older medications are discovered—in the absence of a pharmaceutical company to sponsor large clinical trials—an effective drug may go unnoticed or unprescribed for these nonstandard uses.

Second, it is important to consider the evidence in favor of a drug's benefit. Is it superior to existing drugs? Will it interact with the currently used medications? Do the benefits outweigh the risks? These ques-

> Always consult with a physician before experimenting with new treatments.

tions apply to all alternative treatments, but especially to herbal and other "natural" medicines, where problems with consistent potency and quality are common. The answers to these questions are not yet available for some of these treatments. Always consult with a physician before experimenting with new treatments, and be wary of miracle cures that promise more than the research can prove.

Chapter 12

Preventing
Alzheimer's Disease

Chapter Question:
My aunt has Alzheimer's disease;
what can I do to avoid getting it?

Some of the risk factors for Alzheimer's disease, such as age and genetic factors, cannot be changed, but lifestyle factors, including vitamin intake, diet, exercise, and intellectual and social activity that have a role in one's chances of developing AD can be changed. In addition, medical conditions such as diabetes and hypertension, which may predispose a person toward developing dementia, cannot always be controlled, but the quality of treatment may alter the risk of developing AD. There are *always* choices about care.

RISK FACTORS

A RISK FACTOR IS SOMETHING that increases the chances of developing a medical condition. Risk factors can include the nonmodifiable ones that cannot be prevented, such as age and genetic factors, as well as modifiable ones over which some control can be exerted, such as dietary and lifestyle choices. Risk factors are generally determined by two main types of research study designs: retrospective and prospective. *Retrospective studies* review the records or reports about individuals from the past. *Prospective studies* gather groups of people together and conduct ongoing studies of them into the future.

Retrospective studies are the most common design, because they are easier to conduct and less expensive than prospective studies. For example, an investigator may acquire extensive records of people *with* AD and people *without* AD. The goal is to reconstruct each person's exposure to various factors in the past. Some variables might include the types and quantities of foods eaten; exercise habits; whether and how much a person smoked, drank alcohol, or used certain drugs; the type of environment in which the person lived; and how often the person received health check-ups. Statistical techniques are used to determine if people with AD had significantly more or less exposure to a given factor. Retrospective studies can provide useful information, but when they rely heavily on individual recall (as opposed to medical or school records) they tend to suffer from both positive and negative recall bias. People may have a difficult time remembering certain patterns of behavior over the course of a lifetime. In some cases, the caregiver may answer the questions on behalf of the patient and may unintentionally exaggerate or minimize the person's history with regard to a particular risk factor.

On the other hand, prospective studies of AD risk factors typically start with a group of cognitively normal people and follow them over the course of many years, collecting as much information as possible about them. Eventually, some develop AD and some do not. A careful analysis might reveal differences between the AD group and the non-AD group in various factors. The problem of recall bias is minimized in a prospective study. If the study ends too soon, however, individuals in the non-AD group may go on to develop AD, which would make the original analyses invalid.

When reviewing risk factors, it is important to remember that they are not black and white rules. For example, if you do "X," you will not necessarily develop "Y." All of us can think of a friend or family member who smoked cigarettes her whole life and never developed lung cancer

> **Risk factors are not black and white rules.**

or other smoking-related illnesses. When reviewed across large groups of individuals, however, risk factors stick out like a sore thumb. Genetics, environment, and lifestyle help determine the psychological and medical condition of our bodies. Some influences are more powerful than others, but it is wise to consider your own behavior when modifiable risk factors are identified.

RISK FACTORS FOR ALZHEIMER'S DISEASE

As with any condition, the risk factors for AD can vary in strength and modifiability. For example, rare genetic forms of AD do exist, and a person with one of these rare mutated genes has a 100 percent chance of developing AD if they live long enough. On the other hand, some of the lifestyle risk factors may only minimally increase a person's chances. Table 12-1 lists some nonmodifiable risk factors for developing AD; Table 12-2 lists some modifiable ones. There are varying degrees of support for these factors, with some being firmly established and others having only pre-

Table 12-1: Nonmodifiable Risk Factors for Alzheimer's Disease

1. Older Age
2. Ethnicity
3. Genetics
   a. APP Mutations
   b. Presenilin 1 and 2 Mutations
   c. ApoE4 allele

Table 12.2: Modifiable Risk Factors in Alzheimer's Disease

Dietary
Omega-3 Fatty Acids, Vitamins E and C, B Vitamins

Cardiovascular Risk Factors
Smoking, Diabetes, Hypertension, History of Stroke, Elevated Cholesterol, Statin Use

Lifestyle Factors
Alcohol, Exercise, Amount of Intellectual and Social Activity

Education and General Intelligence

Psychological
Anxious Personality, History of Depression

Hormonal
Estrogen Supplements, Free Testosterone Levels (males)

Head Trauma

liminary evidence supporting their importance. There may also be important interactions among risk factors, but overall there is little understanding regarding the effects of various combinations of risk factors.

Nonmodifiable Risk Factors

Age
The older one gets, the greater the chances are of developing AD. By ages 65–70 years, the prevalence of AD is about 1.5 percent, which translates into 15 people out of 1,000 having the disease. The prevalence approximately doubles with each 5-year increase in age, so that by ages 70–74 years, the prevalence is 3.5 percent; by 75–79 years it is 6.8 percent, and so on until ages 95–99 years when it reaches 44.5 percent. While these numbers show a clear effect of aging on disease, they do not offer an explanation. The interaction of the aging process and the pathologic AD process is under intense investigation, but as of the time of this writing, it is not well understood.

Ethnicity
Some studies have reported higher rates of dementia in ethnic minorities, particularly African-Americans. Other studies that have adjusted the results to account for age, education, and other factors, however, found no significant impact of race on dementia rates. Interestingly, among Asians, the proportion of dementia resulting from vascular disease has increased, which has resulted in a corresponding drop in AD.

Genetics
In general, people who have a parent or sibling with AD have a 3.5-fold higher risk of developing AD themselves, especially if the disease developed relatively early. The risk of developing AD is about 50 percent if both parents developed the presenile form of the disease. Genetics exert

> People who have a parent or sibling with AD have a 3.5-fold higher risk of developing AD.

a strong influence over the expression of pathologic processes, and, in some cases, changes in modifiable risk factors cannot counteract a person's genetic fate.

Three genes have been implicated in causing the rare familial forms of AD. These genes code for the *APP protein*, the *presenilin 1 protein*, and the *presenilin 2 protein*, all of which are involved in the formation of the amyloid peptides (protein chains) that were discussed in Chapter 7. Gene mutations affecting these proteins promote the formation of amyloid plaques, which contributes to the AD process. The study of these dynamics is an important part of AD research, but less than 1 percent of the AD population actually has these gene mutations.

Patients afflicted with one of these rare mutations tend to develop symptoms relatively early, usually in their 40s and 50s, but there are reports of people developing problems in their 30s and even earlier. Every person who inherits one of these genes will develop AD if they survive long enough. There are rather expensive commercially available tests for these genes, and they may be advisable for people with a family history of dementia and relatively early onset AD. (Further information about these tests may be found at www.genetests.org.)

Another important genetic marker is the *ApoE4* gene. *Apolipoprotein E* is one of the proteins involved in cholesterol transport. There have also been reports of complex interactions of the ApoE protein with both the amyloid and tau proteins. There are three major genetic variants (alleles) of this protein, *ApoE2*, *ApoE3*, and *ApoE4*. Each person has two variants of this gene, one from each parent. About 15 to 30 percent of the population has at least one E4 allele, and about 2 percent are *homozygous*—meaning the genes from both parents are the same for the E4 allele. Numerous studies have shown a significantly increased risk of AD in those who have one E4 allele, and a markedly increased risk (up to tenfold) among the few possessing two E4 alleles. The age at onset is also younger among E4 carriers. Conversely, there seems to be a protective effect among those with the E2 allele; whereas the E3 allele is neutral.

Testing for the ApoE genotype is commercially available at a cost of around $250, although its use is under considerable debate. Many people with an E4 allele, even those with two E4 alleles (*homozygotes*), do not develop AD. On the other hand, many people without the E4 allele do develop AD. Consequently, this test is not appropriate for asymptomatic family members concerned with their level of personal risk.

The use of genetic testing as a diagnostic tool is even more controversial. It is clearly not necessary for patients with clinically obvious symptoms. However, in selected cases, in which symptoms are mild or questionable, the presence of an E4 allele does increase the likelihood of AD being present. Since this marker is a risk factor, and it is neither necessary nor sufficient for a person to develop AD, more research is needed regarding how it can be applied clinically. One possible application could be testing patients with mild cognitive impairment (MCI) to see if the ApoE4 allele determines their progression to AD.

Modifiable Risk Factors

Modifiable risk factors are factors over which there is some control. These factors should be viewed as processes that can be changed before the diagnosis of AD. Although it is tempting to do so, it cannot be assumed that because a risk factor may influence the development of AD that alteration of that risk factor will be useful once AD has started to develop. Still, some of these variables are being studied as both a risk factor and a possible treatment intervention, such as vitamin E, but so far none have been proved effective. In addition, some of the modifiable factors listed in Table 12.2 may interact with genetic risk factors in the development of AD.

Dietary Factors

Omega-3 fatty acids are a form of polyunsaturated fats, one of the four basic types of fats the body derives from food. Other types of fat include cholesterol, monounsaturated, and saturated fats. Omega-3 fatty acids are mainly found in cold-water fish, such as salmon or tuna. They have been associated with improved heart health, better cognition in middle-aged adults, and reduced risk of vascular illnesses. With respect to AD, the results have been mixed. Two large-scale studies on fatty acids and AD have come to completely different conclusions. One study reports that the risk of AD was reduced in those consuming fish on average once a week; the other did not find any association with dietary fat intake and AD risk. Future studies are necessary to determine the role of fatty acids in dementia.

The role of antioxidants, such as vitamins E and C, is even more confusing. For example, one study claimed that only dietary vitamin E, not vitamin E supplements, helped to reduce the risk of AD. Another study claimed that vitamin E by itself did nothing, but people who took both vitamin E and C supplements had a reduced risk of developing AD. Yet another study found no association, alone or in combination, of vitamins E and C with AD risk reduction. The reasons for these conflicting results are unclear, but it is probably a safe assumption that the effect on the prevention of AD by antioxidant vitamins is relatively weak, if it exists at all.

Similarly, studies with several of the B Vitamins (B_6, B_{12}, and folic acid) have produced mixed results and conflicting recommendations. The appropriate dose is also undetermined, because some physicians feel only prescription strength supplements will show a benefit. Regardless of the controversies surrounding the specifics of diet and dementia, it is always wise to regularly eat a healthy diet that includes all of the recommended vitamins and minerals. In addition, the use of vitamin supplements is safe and relatively inexpensive.

Cardiovascular Risk Factors

A good rule of thumb is "what is good for the heart is good for the brain." Many of the risk factors for cardiovascular problems may also be involved in cognitive decline and AD later in life. Along the same lines,

> What is good for the heart is good for the brain.

many risk factors for a heart attack are the same as those for a stroke. Stroke is itself a risk factor for dementia. People with diabetes and high blood pressure are more likely to develop dementia. On the other hand, once a person has AD, lowering blood pressure too much may actually worsen cognition, perhaps by decreasing blood flow to the brain.

Smoking is a well-accepted risk factor for cardiovascular disease and stroke, but it is a more controversial dementia risk factor. Several early studies suggested that smoking may actually protect against dementia. These studies did not account for health, wealth, and education, however. Prospective studies show that smokers are at a greater risk for developing dementia and cognitive decline than nonsmokers. For example, a Chinese study of over 2,000 people who were followed prospectively for 2 years found that smokers had more than twice the risk of developing AD or vascular dementia compared to nonsmokers. Furthermore, there was a dose-dependent effect, with heavy smokers having a higher risk than light smokers.

Cholesterol, another important factor in cardiovascular health, appears to be at best, a weak risk factor for AD. Some studies, such as the large-scale Framingham study, have shown no association at all; whereas several smaller studies have claimed a mild statistical increase in risk for AD with higher cholesterol levels.

The strength of the individual contributions of these different risk factors varies by study, but there may be a powerful effect when several are present within the same person. For example, a study led by Rachel Whitmer and colleagues evaluated over 11,000 people who were members of an HMO. They reviewed the detailed health evaluations of everyone aged 40 to 44 during the years 1964 to 1973. About 20 to 40 years later, during the years 1994 to 2003, approximately 885 of these people were diagnosed with dementia. The presence of hypertension, elevated cholesterol, and diabetes at midlife each raised the chances of developing dementia by 20 to 40 percent. Smoking had a borderline association with dementia. However, the odds of being diagnosed with dementia increased by over 250 percent in individuals having all four risk factors. This study shows the impact that multiple risk factors can have on health during a person's life.

Lifestyle Factors
Several large epidemiologic studies have shed light on the complex relationship between alcohol intake and the risk of developing AD. For

example, a study led by Mayeux found that wine (but not beer or liquor) intake of up to three glasses per day was associated with a lower risk of AD, but only in people without the ApoE4 allele. Other studies have also stressed the beneficial effects of low to moderate intake of wine, which is associated with a lower risk of dementia, stroke, and heart disease. On the other hand, higher doses of alcohol are associated with an *increased* risk of dementia. Alcoholics are at significant risk for developing dementia from brain damage caused directly by the alcohol and/or nutritional deficiencies associated with an alcoholic lifestyle.

A second influential lifestyle factor is exercise. Although the benefits of exercise on both physical and mental well-being are well established,

> Exercise affects both brain structure and function.

the specific effects of exercise on the biology of brain function are less understood. Some research has concluded that exercise affects both brain structure and function. In rats, for example, exercise increases the levels of certain growth factors in the hippocampus. Although animal studies do not necessarily parallel human experience, studies of exercise in relationship to AD have provided evidence that:

- A program of regular exercise in midlife is protective against developing AD later in life. Conversely, obesity in midlife increases AD risk.
- Elderly people who exercise regularly are at lower risk of developing AD.
- Exercise can benefit both the AD patient and the caregiver.

It is unclear whether the beneficial effects of exercise are mediated indirectly through lowering the incidence of other diseases, such as hypertension, diabetes, and obesity, or directly through some physiologic effect on brain function, or both. It has also not been determined precisely how much or what type of exercise is best to recommend. Data from the Honolulu Heart Study indicated that even low intensity exercise is beneficial: Elderly men who walked less than a quarter of a mile per day had nearly double the risk of developing dementia compared to those who walked more than 2 miles daily. In addition, further study found that long-term physical activity correlates with better cognitive function in older women. In general, exercise is beneficial, and everyone who does not have some medical contraindication would be better off with a regular exercise program.

Physical exercise is not the only recommended activity for happy, healthy lives. Intellectual and social activity can be just as important in preventing cognitive decline and slowing its progression. Studies have suggested that intellectual activity is protective against AD, regardless of education. For example, a prospective study led by R.S. Wilson used data from the Chicago Health and Aging Project, which is an ongoing study of aging and AD. Over 4,000 residents of South Chicago, aged 65 and older, were interviewed at 3-year intervals over the course of about 5 years. Those who were more intellectually active were less likely to develop AD. For example, those who did crossword puzzles and read books showed less cognitive decline as they aged than those who preferred less cognitively engaging activities, such as watching television. This was true even when considering education, depression, medical conditions, and other influences. In addition to intellectual exercise, several studies have indicated that older people who stay more socially active are less likely to develop AD than their more socially isolated peers.

Education and General Intelligence

Education level was one of the first environmental risk factors identified for AD. People with lower levels of education have higher rates of AD. Although this statement is not disputed, there are several explanations for this risk factor. One theory, called the *synaptic reserve hypothesis*, claims that an educated person has more *synapses* (nerve cell connections) in their brain than a less educated person. Consequently, when a synapse is destroyed by the AD disease process, another one can more easily take its place. A related theory is the *cognitive reserve hypothesis*, which states that highly educated people can better compensate for any loss of abili-

> Highly educated people can better
> compensate for any loss of ability.

ty by using the alternative strategies on tests that they acquired during the course of their education. It is presumed that less educated people lack this flexibility in test-taking strategy.

A fairly different explanation involves the difficulty of diagnosing AD early in highly educated people. The tests used for diagnosis are too easy for them (see Chapter 4). They may score less than they would have before the disease began, but they still score in the normal range. This phenomenon is called *ascertainment bias*. In other words, it is harder to ascertain, or determine, that a highly-educated person has dementia. This bias has been corroborated anatomically by studies showing that for a given Mini-Mental Status Examination (MMSE) score, a person with a college degree will have higher amounts of AD pathology in their brain than a person who dropped out of the fourth grade.

A third theory uses *native intelligence* to explain the links between AD and education. Intelligence, as measured by an *intelligence quotient* (IQ), is highly correlated with achieved educational level. There is also clear evidence for a considerable genetic contribution to intelligence. Some have suggested that higher native intellectual abilities cause both increased educational level and a lowered risk for AD. This also means that the correlation between education and AD risk may be coincidental.

A prospective Dutch study of cognitively normal elderly people showed that a low "DART-IQ" (an estimate of IQ based on reading abilities) was better than years of education at predicting the development of dementia over the 4-year time course of the study. An ongoing prospective study, which measured the intellectual abilities of 2,058 people who were age 15 in 1961, published data in 2004 showing that those with lower intelligence declined more rapidly in memory abilities between the ages of 43 and 53. (In the future, the authors will likely report how many of these individuals develop dementia.) Lastly, the Religious Orders study produced similar results. Nuns who wrote more complex admission essays in their teens were less likely to develop AD decades later. One could postulate that the brighter students wrote the better essays, and whatever brain mechanisms were responsible for their intellectual abilities also protected them from developing the disease.

There may be several factors operating for the observed "protective effect" of education on developing AD. More studies are necessary to reconcile the many possible explanations. Regardless, it is important to keep in mind that having a Ph.D. does not preclude one from developing AD; nor does dropping out of the third grade predestine one towards dementia.

Psychological Stress

There is only one study that specifically reports on the relationship of stress to AD. In the Religious Orders study, people who were more prone to psychologic stress were also more prone to developing AD. It has been postulated that, because stress causes the release of *glucocorticoid* hormones (stress hormones), which in excessive amounts can cause damage to the hippocampus, that perhaps stress predisposes this area of the brain to the AD disease process. In addition to nonspecific stressors, anxiety and depression are associated with an increased risk for AD and may be symptoms of the illness (see Chapter 8).

Hormones

Study of the relationship between hormones and AD has not proved especially fruitful. Estrogen supplements were found to actually increase the risk of AD in women. Testosterone in men has faired slightly better thus far. It is well known that testosterone declines in older males (the "male menopause"), much like estrogen levels decline in older females. There is some evidence that testosterone may reduce levels of β-amyloid and phosphorylated tau (precursor to neurofibrillary tangles). Small clinical studies on testosterone and AD have reported conflicting results. One study from the Baltimore Longitudinal Study of Aging provided evidence that the levels of free testosterone were lower in males who subsequently developed AD. To date, only a few small studies have been published regarding testosterone as a treatment for males with AD. Although these studies have shown some positive results, much larger studies are needed in order to draw firmer conclusions.

Head Injury

It is well known that boxers are prone to develop a kind of dementia called *dementia pugilistica*, a progressive neurologic syndrome characterized by brain damage, psychosis, dementia, personality change, impaired social functioning, and *parkinsonism* (motor problems). Two *meta-analyses* (studies combining the results from several studies) have shown that head trauma sufficient to cause loss of consciousness is associated with a 50 percent greater risk of AD. This effect was only present in males, however. It is speculated that female hormones might be protective to some degree against the deleterious effects of head injury. There is also some evidence that having the ApoE4 allele may interact with head trauma to increase the risk of AD.

A Brief Note on Aluminum and AD

Some years ago, initial studies indicated that there seemed to be a link between the amount of aluminum in the water supply and the risk of developing AD. Furthermore, animal studies showed that aluminum was toxic to neurons. Thus was born the theory that aluminum causes AD. This was one of the very first theories of a cause for AD, and it was widely discussed. Older textbooks and some current popular books on AD still mention it. There were some criticisms of the original studies, however, and subsequent studies cast doubt on the relationship between aluminum intake and the risk of AD. For example, people who used antacids that contained aluminum had no higher risk of developing AD than those who did not. Furthermore, in studies kidney dialysis patients who developed dementia and were exposed to very high levels of aluminum, autopsies of their brains showed different pathologic changes than those seen in AD: No amyloid plaques or neurofibrillary tangles could be found. For these and other reasons, the aluminum theory of AD has lost support, and most researchers have concluded that it is not involved in the disease.

Conclusions about AD Risk Factors

A number of genetic and environmental risk factors for AD have been identified or proposed. Many of these factors are modifiable. The best recommendation to reduce the risk for developing Alzheimer's disease is to follow every mother's advice: Eat a good diet, take your vitamins, do not smoke, drink alcohol in moderation, exercise, do not get stressed out, be happy, and get an education! To tackle the nonmodifiable factors, of course, there is only one thing you can do: Choose your parents wisely.

Chapter 13

Practical Issues for the Patient and Family

Chapter Question:
What about driving, managing finances,
and things like that?

AD patients are at higher risk for motor vehicle accidents. Patients with moderate AD should not drive. Individualized assessment is necessary for patients with mild AD. The patient should designate a family member early in the disease process to take over financial decisions and management. Consultation with a lawyer and obtaining a power of attorney may become necessary.

> AD patients are at higher risk for motor vehicle accidents.

DRIVING

IN 2003, AN ELDERLY DRIVER in California mistook the brake for the gas pedal and plowed into a farmers' market, killing and injuring numerous people. The incident brought national attention to the issue of elderly drivers. Even for nondemented older adults, general slowing of reaction time and relatively impaired vision and hearing can increase the risk of accidents. Dementia is also accompanied by cognitive problems and impaired judgment, further elevating the risk of a driving accident. In particular, AD patients are at risk for driving errors that can cause accidents, such as getting lost, slower reaction times, making the wrong decision in a complex traffic situation, and driving the wrong way on a one-way street.

Driving regulations regarding AD vary from state to state and country to country. In California, for example, doctors are required by law to report people with dementia to the Department of Motor Vehicles (DMV). The DMV subsequently decides, on a case by case basis, whether driving privileges should be restricted or eliminated. In other countries, programs concerning elderly drivers have produced varying results. In Finland, regular recertifications of fitness to drive are required for the elderly. Unfortunately, studies showed no reduction in the number of older people dying because of car crashes, but there was an increase in elderly persons dying as pedestrians and cyclists. In Australia, a national law requires a person to inform the local drivers' license authority of any condition that may affect safety, including dementia. People with such conditions undergo an on-road driving test with a specially trained occupational therapist, in addition to a driving history, medical history, hearing and vision tests, and a general physical examination. Among dementia patients in Australia, 30 percent pass and are reevaluated annually. Another 30 percent have driving restricted to certain distances and/or times of day, and 40 percent have their licenses cancelled.

In 2001, the American Academy of Neurology issued a "practice parameter" stating that all patients with clinically definite dementia should not drive. Since that time, however, studies evaluating the driving performance and safety over time in AD patients have shown that:

- Driving is not significantly impaired in the MCI stage.
- About half of the patients with mild AD are still reasonably safe drivers, but half are not.
- All moderate stage AD patients are clearly unsafe on the road.

So although moderate patients should not drive, and MCI patients will likely be unimpaired, mild AD patients need more extensive evaluation. Decisions about driving must be individualized, and family input is critical. If a family member has observed unsafe driving behaviors, such as running stop signs and poorly judged lane changes, then it is time for the patient to give up her license. In doubtful cases, the patient may consider taking a DMV driving test. It is critical that periodic re-evaluations be performed of mildly demented patients who are still considered safe drivers, because studies have documented a decline in driving performance over time in AD.

An interesting Italian study headed by Dr. E. Uc compared the driving performance of mild AD patients to normal elderly patients of the same age using a specially outfitted car. Just before the driving test, the subjects were given a set of verbal directions that they had to repeat correctly twice, mimicking a situation in which someone is told how to get somewhere. The AD patients made significantly more safety errors, incorrect turns, and tended to get lost more often than the control subjects. The authors noted that some of the AD patients performed quite well, and patients who were relatively familiar with the area where the driving test was done performed better than those who were driving in unfamiliar territory. This study again highlights the importance of individualized driving assessment in early AD and it hints that if driving is confined to familiar routes it is less likely that the patient will make safety errors.

Although safety is the most important concern, the loss of independence that results from losing driving privileges is significant. This new dependence on others can lead to anger, frustration, and feelings of

> Driving concerns should be handled compassionately.

worthlessness in the patient, and driving concerns should be handled compassionately. If family members do not feel that the patient will voluntarily give up driving or respond to gentle coaxing, it may be helpful for the physician to simply instruct the patient that he cannot drive. Family members may even need to meet with the doctor privately to discuss their concerns.

If family members find that strict orders from the physician are not enough to keep the patient from driving, more drastic measures must be tried. Consider confiscating keys or parking the car out of sight. If the urge to drive seems to be triggered by the sight of the family car, try selling it and replacing it with a different vehicle.

MANAGING FINANCES

Over the course of Alzheimer's disease, the patient will become less able to manage the family and business finances. Unfortunately, family members may not realize this until, for example, the utility company shuts off the power, or stacks of unpaid bills are discovered along with a checkbook that is not up-to-date and contains gross calculation errors. A study of financial abilities in mild cognitive impairment (MCI) and AD led by H.R. Griffith found that, even in MCI, patients suffered mild deficits in financial capacity. In mild AD patients, these deficits were more pronounced and included more activities. Only the simplest measures, such as recognizing coins, were completely spared.

This study emphasizes the need to get help early in the illness. Arrangements should be made for someone to help with and then eventually take over financial tasks. This may be easier said than done. Fiercely independent and stubborn individuals may insist on managing family or business assets even when presented with recent losses or miscalculations. Conversely, the patient's involvement in complex activities can be healthy and should be encouraged. While there are no easy answers for this situation, family members can attempt to reason with the patient and seek advice from long-trusted friends and business advisors. An extreme solution is to take legal action to declare the person incompetent and obtain a power of attorney. This may result in severe stress and hostility, however, not only for the patient, but for other family members who may not agree with this approach. Therefore, it is important for all concerned parties, including the patient, to openly share in the discussion.

Of course, there is no limit to the complexity of situations that can arise when, for example, a patient has multiple children from different marriages, or when a wealthy, demented widower hooks up with (in the eyes of his children) a gold-digging bombshell. The resulting ethical and legal dilemmas can truly test the wisdom of the finest philosophers and judges.

At a minimum, any person who is newly diagnosed with dementia should have his financial affairs reviewed by an accountant and/or attorney, or by a family member, as soon as possible to make sure everything

> Consult with a knowledgeable financial
> planner.

is in order and that there is a system in place for the bills to be paid. It is also important to formulate a long-term financial plan for both the family and the patient. The cost of care for an AD patient is high, with the Alzheimer's Association estimating that families will spend, on average, $175,000 throughout the course of the disease. Therefore, it is critically important to consult with a knowledgeable financial planner, accountant, and/or attorney to devise a strategy for the future.

WILLS

Just as financial affairs must be reviewed early in the illness, so must the patient's will. In order to craft a will, the patient must be competent to communicate his wishes. A decline in cognition, although often gradual, can occur suddenly. If the patient is fully competent to direct the will, the family members can be comfortable that his wishes will be fulfilled. The patient's will is not the only consideration, however. The primary caregiver should also construct his will so that the instructions are clear in the event he dies before the patient.

DURABLE POWER OF ATTORNEY

Someone must be chosen in advance to make good decisions for a person with AD, because they will eventually become unable to make decisions for themselves. A simple *power of attorney*, which gives a designated person the authority to manage the finances, property, and so forth for another person, becomes void when the person becomes incompetent. This is impractical for people with AD. Another alternative is the *durable power of attorney*, which remains in place when a person becomes mentally incapacitated. If the person with AD has someone they can trust, it is recommended that this person be assigned a durable power of attorney, particularly if there is some degree of family discord, or if no close relative is able to undertake the responsibility. In addition, there is the *durable power of attorney for health care*, with the designated person's responsibilities limited to health care decisions. An attorney is required for the preparation of each of these documents, and the patient must be competent to sign them. If the patient becomes incompetent before these tasks can be completed, a conservatorship may become necessary. This involves court proceedings, including a hearing by a judge.

SAFETY CONSIDERATIONS

Once an AD patient has moved from the mild phase of the illness to the moderate phase, he may be at risk for wandering behaviors. All moderate AD patients should wear a medical identification bracelet to ensure their safety. These can be obtained through a local chapter of the

> Moderate AD patients should wear a medical identification bracelet to ensure their safety.

Alzheimer's Association. More futuristic methods, such as the implantation of microchips that contain medical history and identifying information, and have the ability to locate persons using global position satellite (GPS) technology, are now available through some companies and will likely become widespread. All kinds of gizmos and gadgets, such as automatic electronic pill dispensers, are available not only for AD patients, but to help all elderly people maintain an independent lifestyle; www.age-in-place.com is a Web site where such products can be viewed. Physical means of preventing the patient from going outside may become necessary; for example, installing a deadbolt that requires a key on the inside of the front door, or having an alarm installed on the door.

Common sense home safety considerations include keeping medications and potentially toxic substances in a safe place, using night-lights, having emergency phone numbers and contact information in plain sight, keeping fire extinguishers and a first aid kit handy, and making sure that smoke alarms work. An excellent book for an in-depth analysis of this topic is: *The Complete Guide to Alzheimer's Proofing Your Home*, by M.L. Warner (Purdue University Press, 2000). There are also numerous Web sites that provide helpful safety tips for AD patients and caregivers, including www.alzheimers-illinois.org/tips/safety.html.

TRAVELING AND VACATIONS

Taking a vacation with an AD patient rarely proves to be restful for a caregiver. If the primary caregiver needs a relaxing vacation, then it is best to arrange for someone else to care for the patient. If the patient will be traveling, extra caution must be observed, particularly once the moderate stages of AD have been reached. Separation and getting lost in an unfamiliar environment is a real possibility. Be sure that in addition to a medic alert bracelet the patient carries caregiver contact information, lodging information, a list of medications, and emergency contacts. Bring familiar pictures or items from home to display in the hotel room, which can help reorient the person. Additional confusion and perhaps unexpected behavioral reactions are possible when the AD patient is brought into a new place with strangers. Consider planning a short trip first before attempting longer stays away from home. Also, avoid planning too many activities and leave adequate rest time between them. In the event that an AD patient must travel alone, you should pay to have an escort, especially if a change of planes is required. Even here, problems may occur. In March of 2004, an AD patient was lost by the escort at an airport while awaiting a connecting flight. Fortunately, he was found a few hours later several miles away at a bus station, but this incident highlights the fact that traveling alone can be a dangerous proposition for an AD patient.

CONCLUDING REMARKS

Caring for an Alzheimer's patient can be demanding and unpredictable. The more prepared the family is, the fewer the surprises. By keeping the person's home and travel environments safe, the caregiver can reduce accidents, minimize confusion and agitation, and encourage the appropriate level of independence. In addition, if family and business finances are secure, and strategies are in place for later stages of the illness, the patient and caregiver can avoid circumstances that could compromise care or eliminate choices.

Transition of Care

Chapter Question:
How do we know when it is time for a nursing home?

In the final stages of Alzheimer's disease, patient care often becomes too difficult for a loved one to manage without professional help. The caregiver may consider moving the patient to an assisted-living facility while some skills are still preserved. Care provided by a skilled nursing home or hospice may become necessary in the terminal phase. Chapter 14 reviews some of the factors affecting nursing home placement, as well as procedures that may be recommended toward the end of the patient's life to improve comfort.

THE DECISION TO UTILIZE PROFESSIONAL HELP

AS A CAREGIVER, you have loved your spouse and provided round-the-clock care as she has become progressively demented and less independent. The demands on your physical, financial, emotional, and spiritual resources have grown tremendously, and you often feel stressed

> Consider getting outside help.

and exhausted, and sometimes angry and depressed. At this point, you realize that you must consider getting outside help.

Initially, a part-time nurse's aide may provide enough relief so that the patient can remain at home. As the disease worsens, professional help may become necessary. The decision to move a loved one to a nursing home is certainly one of the most difficult decisions that must be made. Circumstances vary greatly, making this a highly individualized decision.

When weighing the costs and benefits, many factors need to be considered, some unique to the caregiver, some belonging to the patient. For example, caregivers with physical limitations or who have full-time jobs are more likely to need professional help sooner than relatively healthy, retired caregivers. In addition, the caregiver may need more assistance if the patient regularly displays agitation, aggression, nighttime behaviors, and incontinence. Finally, financial affairs and the availability of quality care also strongly influence placement decisions.

Choosing an Appropriate Facility

The Medicare Web site, www.medicare.gov/Nursing/Overview.asp, allows visitors to search for Medicare-approved nursing facilities within specific geographic areas. It provides the address, phone number, number of beds, type of ownership, and whether or not the facility is located within a hospital. Details regarding quality measures, inspection results, and staffing are also available. The inspection information includes the nature of any deficiencies that have been discovered and their relative risk. The homes are required to develop specific plans to correct deficiencies. These plans are available upon request directly from the facility.

A free referral service is offered through the Web site, www.aplace formom.com, or by calling 1-877-666-3239. Consumers are offered personalized assistance from their assigned family advisor. Many Web sites provide similar services (enter "Alzheimer's nursing home" on any of the large search engines, such as Yahoo or Google). The Alzheimer's Association publishes a booklet entitled *Selecting a Nursing Home with a Dedicated Dementia Unit* that can help guide you in your search. When a prospective home is identified, arrange a tour. Consider making multiple visits at different times to observe the ongoing activities and how the residents interact with the staff. Finally, ask a friend or family member to visit as well. It never hurts to have a second opinion.

Assisted Living versus Nursing Homes

Approximately 5 percent of elderly Americans live in nursing facilities, and it is estimated that at least 45 percent of these are demented. Another 5 percent live in assisted-living or board and care homes, of which 30 percent are estimated to be demented. There has been substantial growth in the assisted-living industry in the last 10 years, and many facilities now include special features designed to fit the needs of the cognitively impaired. These are called *assisted-living dementia care facilities* (ALDC), or their nursing level dementia care counterpart, *NLDC units*.

An ALDC facility has several advantages over a regular assisted-living home. The staff in an ALDC facility has had special training in dementia care skills and provides a range of activities designed for demented people. The number of residents is limited, ideally to 20, but it may be up to 35. The exit doors are locked by a digital key pad; lighting levels are kept high; and there is easy access to an outdoor space designed for safety and surrounded by a protective fence. These units typically include measures that can adjust the amount of sensual stimulation via noise, lighting, and odor controls. They should provide access to natural daylight, and be designed with contrasting colors that can aid in the location of handrails and toilets, while also taking into account the fact that elderly individuals may have trouble seeing blue, violet, purple, and red. NLDC facilities are somewhat similar to ALDC, but they focus on simpler activities and provide more extensive nursing services.

These specialized dementia programs are often located in small, independently operated homes, multiple small homes with joint administration, or larger programs that may cater exclusively to dementia patients or are part of a multilevel facility. Many such facilities incorporate both assisted-living and nursing level care. Assisted-living settings are appropriate for people who are ambulatory and can carry out the activities of daily living with minimal supervision. Nursing level facilities are designed for those who require active assistance with feeding, toileting, and bathing. For the most advanced patients, for example, GDS level 7 (see Chapter 4), additional measures are necessary to accommodate their needs, such as stronger odor control, close supervision for thermal comfort, and indirect lighting.

Hospice

For a patient still at home but in the advanced stages of AD (GDS 6 or 7), hospice care may be an alternative to nursing level care facilities.

> Hospice services focus on comfort rather than treatment.

Hospice services focus on comfort rather than treatment and are appropriate for advanced terminally ill patients. A hospice evaluation involves social workers, nurses, bereavement counselors, and a hospice physician, but will only be conducted when a doctor certifies in writing that the patient has less than 6 months to live. Medicare will often cover hospice services, which can be continued even if home care becomes unmanageable and a nursing home is required. Hospice can be a very positive experience for both patient and family.

Financing Care

Assisted living or nursing care can be expensive, approximately $40,000 per year. Medicaid programs typically cover facility care, although families may have to spend a significant portion of their resources before becoming eligible. If assets are transferred into another person's name 30 months before placement, however, they will not be considered when the patient applies for Medicaid. Unfortunately, because of the differences in reimbursement rates, many facilities limit the number of patients who are on Medicaid or who will require it. Consultation with an experienced financial advisor well in advance of the anticipated need for a nursing home is strongly recommended. For example, the advisor may suggest an insurance policy that will help cover the cost of facility care, although the premiums are often expensive and few people utilize this alternative. In addition, the State Health Insurance Assistance Program, which is available in each state, has counselors who can provide advice regarding any government funding that may be available. Phone numbers for each state can be found on the Medicare Web site.

PREDICTING TIME TO NURSING HOME PLACEMENT

A study headed by Y. Stern followed AD patients for up to 7 years until they either died or entered a care facility. For mild AD patients who were around 74 years old, the most likely duration until nursing home placement was about 28 months. By 47 months into the study, 75 percent of the participants in this age group were in a care facility. Stern and colleagues later conducted an investigation that concluded the risk of nursing home placement is related to the rate of cognitive decline. A substantial decline in test scores over the course of a year from diagnosis may indicate that out-of-home placement will soon become necessary.

If the rate of cognitive decline is associated with time to nursing home placement, then will the drugs that slow the rate of cognitive decline also prolong the time to placement? The first major investigation into this question was published by David Geldmacher and colleagues. This study followed patients who had originally volunteered for clinical trials of the drug Aricept®. It compared those who dropped out of the first study, those who were treated with placebo, and those who did not participate in the subsequent longer study with patients who continued on into the longer study. In general, they found that the longer the patients had been exposed to Aricept®, the longer it took before they entered a nursing home. Criticisms of this study have emerged, however.

A second study, conducted by Simu Thomas, found similar results. This study compared the rate of nursing home placement of over 2,500 patients categorized into three groups: 1) patients taking Exelon® (rivastigmine); 2) patients taking Aricept® (donepezil); and 3) untreated patients. The untreated patients were three times as likely as the treated patients to be placed in a nursing home.

The results of the AD2000 trial, which were published in June 2004 in *Lancet*, were contrary to the studies mentioned above. This study had the merit of being a double-blind, placebo-controlled trial of donepezil. Over 500 AD patients (with an average MMSE of 20) were enrolled and followed over a period of several years. There was no difference in the rate of nursing home placement in those taking Aricept® versus those on placebo. However, several criticisms of this study make the results questionable. For example, at the end of 3 years, only 20 people remained in the study. Also, the study protocol called for a 6-week washout period after every 48 weeks of treatment. Based on previous studies of donepezil, this amount of time without treatment is sufficient to eliminate all benefit from the drug.

At this time, although there is considerable evidence suggesting that the cholinesterase drugs may prolong time to placement in a nursing home, there are not enough studies to warrant a firm consensus. It is unlikely that another long-term, double-blind trial will be possible to conduct, because it would require some patients being deprived of an approved treatment for a period of possibly many years.

END-OF-LIFE CARE ISSUES

The appropriate levels of care for people with end-stage dementia involve both medical and ethical considerations. The caregiver is often faced with the difficult choice of giving permission for a therapeutic procedure that may be uncomfortable for the patient and will likely prolong the process of dying, or denying the treatment. The caregiver may feel that by refusing permission she will somehow be responsible for the earlier death of the patient.

For example, *gastrostomy tubes* may become an option when patients lose the ability to eat on their own. These tubes are surgically placed by a gastroenterologist directly into the stomach. The patient is fed through the tube with a specially prepared liquid food, such as Ensure®. An alternative to this procedure is a *nasogastric feeding tube*, which is inserted through the nose and down into the stomach. Unfortunately, they can only be used for a few weeks, because the tube tends to erode the lining of the nostril. While it seems cruel to let someone die of starvation, a study by L.M. Murphy and T.O. Lipman concluded that there was, in fact, no difference in survival (average 2 months) between those who received a gastrostomy tube and those who did not.

The second difficult choice involves the decision to resuscitate. Performing life-saving procedures on a dementia patient whose heart has stopped beating is virtually always a futile effort. In cases where the "Code Blue" is successful in reviving the heart muscle, there is usually severe and irreversible brain damage. Thus, resuscitation in this setting generally serves only to prolong the suffering of the family and perhaps the patient. If the patient and family have decided against resuscitation, then paperwork should be completed for an advance directive called a "Do Not Resuscitate (DNR)" order.

ASSESSING PAIN IN ADVANCED AD

A major concern of caregivers is that their loved one is in pain. Although this can be difficult to assess in those who cannot speak, pain can be expressed in other ways. Behaviors such as vocalizations (whimpering, groaning, or crying), and facial expressions of tension, fear, or grimacing

> Physical changes must be noted and addressed.

are clear signs of pain. More subtle signs include changes in body language, changes in usual patterns of behavior, and physiologic changes such as perspiration or pallor. Physical changes, such as skin tears, arthritis, pressure sores, and areas of previous trauma, must be noted and addressed.

There are very few studies on the frequency and severity of pain in advanced AD patients. One study, lead by E. Scherder, suggests that AD patients experience less intense pain during daily activities and show a decrease in the emotional aspect of pain, such as depression related to pain, compared to elderly non-AD adults. In addition, the AD patients reported that pain had less of an impact on their quality of life than the non-AD group. A second study, by J.T. van der Steen, found that pain in AD is sometimes more related to secondary illnesses, such as pneumonia.

IMMEDIATE EFFECTS OF PATIENT DEATH ON THE CAREGIVER

An article published by Richard Shulz and colleagues investigated the experience of caregivers in the year prior to patient death and in the 3 months postmortem. Over half of 200 caregivers reported spending at least 46 hours per week helping patients with the basic activities of daily living and that they felt they were "on duty" 24 hours a day. Many had to end or reduce employment because of caretaking demands. Approximately one-fourth of the patients were placed in facility care during the year prior to their death. Almost three-fourths of the caregivers felt relief when the patient's death occurred, and over 90 percent believed that death also came as a relief to the patient. In addition, caregivers proved to be remarkably resilient, with levels of depression declining substantially within 3 months after the patient's demise.

The journey with a patient suffering a progressive illness is unarguably a complicated one, although careful preparation can eliminate the need to make several difficult decisions under less than optimal circumstances. Community and medical resources can help the patient's transition from suffering to peace occur with comfort and compassion.

Chapter 15

Care for
the Caregiver

Chapter Question:
What can a caregiver do to stay healthy?

The role of caregiver can be extremely stressful. Acquiring education regarding the Alzheimer's disease process, learning strategies to deal with problematic behaviors, utilizing the resources in your community, and even successful medical management of the AD patient can help you become a more effective and healthy caregiver.

CAREGIVERS: THE UNSUNG HEROES OF ALZHEIMER'S DISEASE

INDIVIDUALS ARE OFTEN FORCED to embrace the role of caregiver just as they are anticipating a part of their lives that should include less formal work, more time with loved ones, and plans for travel and leisure. Although grief and a sense of injustice are common upon receiving the initial diagnosis, families are eventually able to overcome these obstacles and move toward "living with Alzheimer's." Family members provide invaluable assistance in coping with the everyday complications of life with an AD patient. Their sacrifice is not always without personal loss, however.

Caregivers work tirelessly to meet the physical, medical, and psychological needs of their loved ones, but may experience emotional, physical, and even financial difficulties of their own. Stress, depression, and social isolation are not uncommon among caregivers of a person with a chronic illness. Managing medical care, prescriptions, and therapy can be scary, and sometimes confusing. Some caregivers are forced to take over the financial and legal matters of the family, a role they may not be comfortable assuming. In addition, caregivers must keep up with their own doctor visits, medicines, and possibly illnesses. The role of caregiver is by no means simple or effortless. For those who have accepted this role, this chapter is devoted to helping you take care of yourself and improve your skills as an effective caregiver to an AD patient.

STEPS TO EFFECTIVE CAREGIVING

Step One

Table 15-1 outlines six steps that can help someone become a better caregiver. Each step includes a simple rule that in practice may not be so easy. The first step: "Forewarned is forearmed!" recommends that you educate yourself regarding the course of AD and the expectations for

> Educate yourself regarding the course of AD.

medical care, personality changes, cognitive functions, and day-to-day activities. Although you may not have wanted to go back to school at this point in your life, there are many practical, scientific, and even humorous resources for caregivers and patients with AD.

All major bookstores carry books on AD that are aimed at the general public. The current selection includes titles such as the classic *The*

Table 15-1: Steps to Effective Caregiving

STEP 1: Forewarned is forearmed!

STEP 2: Get appropriate medical care for your loved one.

STEP 3: Make sure YOU are okay!

STEP 4: Plan ahead!

STEP 5: Share the burden.

STEP 6: Join a support group.

36-Hour Day by Nancy Mace and Peter Rabins; *The Mayo Clinic on Alzheimer's Disease* by the Mayo Clinic; and *Alzheimer's for Dummies* by Patricia Smith, Mary Kenan, Mark Kunik, and Leeza Gibbons. Although there is some overlap in the information presented, each of these books contains unique information and tips that many will find helpful. In addition, online resources number in the tens of thousands. The Resource section lists some of the most helpful Web sites. We strongly encourage caregivers to check out these sites; each will have useful information as well as links to other quality AD Web sites. If you do not have Internet access in your home, any major library should have both the computers and the personnel to help you.

Step Two

"Get appropriate medical care for your loved one" simply means that the better the medical care for the patient, the less the caregiver has to do. There is mounting evidence that the treatment of AD with one of the medications discussed in Chapter 9 also helps the caregiver. Studies with each of the cholinesterase inhibitors has shown that caregivers of patients on medication suffer less subjective stress and devote less time to caregiving activities compared with caregivers of untreated patients.

For example, a study led by Howard Feldman compared Aricept® to placebo in patients with moderate to severe AD over a 24-week period. *Activities of daily living* (ADLs) were assessed using standard scales, and caregivers completed a *Caregiver Stress Scale* in addition to recording the time spent assisting patients. At the start of the study, there were no differences in the patients or caregivers between the Aricept® and placebo group. At the end of the study, both groups had declined somewhat in ADL, but the placebo group had worsened significantly more than the Aricept® group. Consequently, the Aricept® caregivers spent about 52 minutes less per day assisting loved ones and reported significantly less stress. In a similar study with a newer drug, Namenda®, investigators estimated that caregivers spent about 50 hours less per month with moderate to severe AD patients compared with the control group. Last, as discussed in Chapter 9, some of the behaviors seen in AD patients that

> Caregiver stress can be relieved to some extent by medications taken by the person with AD.

can further exacerbate caregiver stress can be relieved to some extent by various antidepressant and antipsychotic medications.

Although these results are encouraging, average relief of an hour per day may not put a significant dent in 24-hour care. Often caregivers report little, if any, changes with medication. Until better treatments are available, however, a little relief is better than no relief.

Step Three

As the AD patient's primary source of daily physical and emotional care, you cannot be an effective caregiver if you are not healthy. Step three: "Make sure that YOU are okay!" should be followed with respect to both emotional and physical well-being. Table 15-2 outlines some signs of caregiver stress. Get help if you are experiencing any of these symptoms. Ask your physician for a recommendation, seek out a support group, or enlist the help of a counselor.

Caregivers of patients with chronic illnesses are at risk for depression. Studies indicate that, on average, about one-third of caregivers of AD patients suffer significant symptoms of depression. In addition to the expected stress and occasional social isolation encountered while caring for an ill person, certain characteristics of both the patient and the care-

---

Table 15-2: Signs of Caregiver Stress

- Emotional symptoms, such as depression, guilt, or anger
- Sleep problems
- Feelings of excessive fatigue
- Feeling that you have no time for yourself
- Feeling isolated and alone
- Less contact with friends and family members
- Increased use of alcohol and medications "for nerves"

giver have been shown to increase the risk of caregiver depression. According to a study by Kenneth Covinsky and colleagues, patients who had behavioral and emotional disturbances, especially anger and aggression, and those with less preserved ADL skills, were more likely to have depressed caregivers. Low income caregivers and those who spent the most time caring for their loved one were more likely to suffer from depression. These findings reinforce the idea that one way of helping the caregiver is to treat the patient. Medications that alleviate some of the emotional and behavioral problems, and those that improve ADL skills, will likely reduce the risk of depression in caregivers.

Step Four

Step four: "Plan ahead!" can save you and your family from having to make difficult choices during distressing times, as well as give the patient a chance to contribute to key decisions. Chapter 13 reviewed the importance of putting financial, legal, and insurance affairs in order. It is also necessary to anticipate new transportation arrangements for when driving becomes unsafe and to discuss assisted-living or nursing home options with your loved one. You will have time to make informed decisions if you start these discussions early. You may even want to consult an eldercare attorney for advice.

Step Five

As AD progresses, the degree of responsibility, time, and effort that the caregiver must provide increases substantially. Eventually there comes a time when it is almost impossible to do the job alone. Step five reminds you to "Share the burden." Asking for help from family, friends, and neighbors can help keep you healthy and possibly extend the period of time before assisted living becomes a necessity. Take some time off to do something you have always enjoyed. Take a nap, or just get some help with shopping and meal preparation. Have a family meeting and be honest with each other. It may be difficult for some, especially children, to realize that you need help. If family members cannot give enough, check with your local Alzheimer's Association about the availability of daycare programs or volunteer sitters (24-hour help line: 1-800-272-3900). Finally, an effective solution may be to hire a home health worker or nurse's aide to provide respite care and help with household chores.

Step Six

Regardless of how well informed you are, how many books on AD you have read, and how many caregiver tips you have memorized, most of the time you are going to have to develop solutions that are as unique

> The support and advice of other caregivers can be invaluable.

as your situation. The last step recommends that you: "Join a support group." Get help from the people in the trenches. The support and advice of other caregivers can be invaluable. Your local Alzheimer's Association chapter can provide details on such meetings or assist you in starting one of your own. There are even on-line chat rooms for AD caregivers that often host specific chat times for people to get together and share their stories and problems. Although this advice may not be professional, guaranteed, or even always accurate, you may find wise, practical suggestions that you can only get from experienced caregivers. These on-line forums can also provide emotional support, especially if attending meetings of a local support group is difficult or inconvenient. Suggestions for dealing with problems in the activities of daily living are listed in Tables 15-3 and 15-4. But do not forget to ask for help, and be creative.

Table 15-3: Suggestions for Help with Activities of Daily Living

1. Getting Dressed
   - Don't rush your loved one; be flexible with their clothing choices
   - Use comfortable and simple clothing, such as shirts with buttons in the front, which are easier to put on than pullovers
   - If your loved one does not want to change clothes, use clothing that can be worn both day and night
   - Sometimes people with AD prefer to wear layers of clothes; do not worry, they will take some off if they get too hot
2. Eating
   - Snacks between meals can help with weight gain
   - Reduce distractions, such as television during mealtimes
   - Play soft music
   - Prepare food so that it can go directly from the plate to the mouth
3. Bathing
   - Set the water heater to 120 degrees to avoid burns
   - Make sure there are nonslip adhesives on the floor
   - Consider installing grab bars in the bathtub
   - Help the person feel in control whenever possible
   - Coach your loved one through each step
4. Using the Bathroom
   - Keep the bathroom door open and a light on at night
   - Keep track of how often they use the bathroom
   - Help them get there ahead of time to avoid accidents

Table 15-4: Ten Absolute Guidelines for Alzheimer's Care

1. Never argue, instead, agree
2. Never reason, instead, divert
3. Never shame, instead, distract
4. Never lecture, instead, reassure
5. Never say remember, instead, reminisce
6. Never say I told you, instead, repeat
7. Never refuse a request, instead, plan an activity they are capable of doing
8. Never command or demand, instead, encourage and praise
9. Never condescend, instead, encourage and praise
10. Never force, instead, reinforce

Chapter 16

The Future of Alzheimer's Research and Treatment

Chapter Question:
Is there hope for the future?

The coming years will hold major advances on three fronts in the fight against Alzheimer's disease: 1) understanding the underlying causes of AD; 2) detection and diagnosis; and 3) treatment. Physicians and researchers are optimistic that some-day there will be a cure, but it is critical that the public support and participate in research efforts to find that cure.

ADVANCES IN THE FIELD OF ALZHEIMER'S DISEASE

THE PATIENTS, FAMILIES, AND CAREGIVERS who experience the devastation associated with Alzheimer's disease may feel isolated and helpless in the face of such an intimidating illness. They may be frustrated and

> Researchers and physicians are determined to improve the methods of detection and treatment of AD.

angry at having to experience this hardship with seemingly no hope for a cure. The newest drugs seem to make only small differences compared to the dramatic changes that patients must endure. However, researchers and physicians are determined to improve the methods of detection and treatment of AD.

Advances in Understanding the Causes of AD

In Chapter 7, we reviewed the progress that has been made in understanding the basic pathology of AD. The major features of an AD brain—atrophy and the presence of amyloid plaques and neurofibrillary tangles, are readily recognized upon autopsy. A deeper understanding of AD depends upon understanding the relationship between these pathologic findings. What causes the plaques and tangles to form? Do the amyloid and tau proteins interact? Why are only certain areas of the brain vulnerable to the AD process? How does the disease spread in the brain? Researchers are striving to create techniques that can help answer these questions. Improved animal models of AD will likely be a key feature of research advances.

There is a conceptual revolution in progress, not only in the field of AD, but in how scientists and doctors think of neurodegenerative diseases in general—diseases such as frontotemporal dementia (FTD), Parkinson's, Huntington's, ALS (Lou Gehrig's disease), and many other lesser known diseases characterized by progressive loss of nervous system function. Many of these diseases have a key similarity to AD: abnormal protein processing. We have seen that the leading theory of the cause of AD involves abnormal processing of a certain protein, the APP. Abnormal processing of another protein, α-synuclein, is a key feature of the formation of the Lewy bodies that are found in Parkinson's *and* in Lewy body dementia. Many cases of FTD are associated with abnormal tau protein. Each of these diseases has a key protein that is different from the others, in which abnormal *aggregation* (sticking together) of the protein occurs. These protein aggregates appear to be toxic to the cell. There are a number of biochemical similarities between the abnormal tau protein in FTD and the mutated α-synuclein involved in some cases of Parkinson's. In fact, each can interact with the other and enhance their toxicity. Thus, what is learned about one protein may have implications for others. Indeed, on the clinical level, doctors are starting to regard Parkinson's and Alzheimer's almost as a disease continuum, with dementia with Lewy bodies and AD with parkinsonian-like features as intermediate states between the two extremes of Parkinson's and AD.

Another area of investigation uses *DNA microarray analysis* to study the expression of thousands of genes at the same time. Studies of diseases such as AD and FTD are being undertaken to discover which genes are overactive and which are underactive. Different diseases have different patterns of gene expression. This technique is a shortcut to help identify the genes and their proteins that may be involved in a given disease.

Advances in Diagnosis

As both preventive and symptomatic treatments for AD continue to multiply, it will become increasingly important to identify people with mild cognitive impairment (MCI) and early AD. In fact, if an effective preventive treatment is found, identifying people in the presymptomatic phase, when the AD pathology has already started but is not advanced enough to produce any detectable symptoms, will become just as important as it is now for other serious illnesses, such as cancer. There is widespread acceptance of screening mammograms, colonoscopies, and blood tests for the detection of breast, colon, and prostate cancer, respectively. Ultimately, screening for AD will become a part of regular health checkups. There is a strong demand for an inexpensive, noninvasive, and reliable test for AD. The following areas offer the most promise:

Positron emission tomography (PET) can help diagnose AD, often showing decreased activity in the temporal and parietal areas. A substance has been developed that binds to brain amyloid, which can then subsequently be detected on PET scanning. Some of the details in using this test require fine-tuning, including confirmation that this approach will be specific for detecting AD as opposed to other forms of dementia. It could also be used for monitoring the course of the disease and evaluating response to therapy. If developed sufficiently, this technique may be able to detect presymptomatic AD. At the 9th International Conference on Alzheimer's Disease and Related Disorders presented by the Alzheimer's Association, results were announced regarding a small study using this new technique in MCI patients. This study that provided evidence that many MCI patients do, in fact, have increased amounts of amyloid in their brains. PET scans can also be customized to examine various biochemical parameters. In another example, Dr. Rik Vandenberghe and colleagues performed a very interesting study of amnestic MCI patients using a special chemical to highlight the cholinesterase enzyme. Compared to normal elderly subjects, the MCI patients had decreased cholinesterase activity in the left deep temporal lobe, an area of the brain that is important for short-term memory (see Chapter 3). The lower level of this enzyme implies that there is a deficit in the acetylcholine system in this area in MCI patients. This is consistent with the notion that MCI represents early AD, because this is the same area of the brain where the AD process often begins.

Conventional magnetic resonance imaging (MRI) and computed tomography (CT) have been used for ruling out other diagnoses when AD is suspected. Advances in computer software allow these images to be represented in ways that could be useful for AD diagnosis. For example, researchers using software that can measure the volume of the brain regions affected early in AD, such as the hippocampus, have been able to show shrinkage in these areas as the disease progresses. Other software modifications, such as functional magnetic resonance imaging (fMRI), reveal how much oxygen is being used in certain parts of the brain while people are engaged in various cognitive tasks. If AD causes local changes in blood oxygenation, this procedure may become important in the near future.

Although there is great interest and hope that a biomarker will prove reliable for confirming the presence of AD, it is likely that doctors will still be reliant on mental status tests for the next several years.

> Identification of the most reliable dementia screening test is of great importance.

Therefore, identification of the briefest, most easily used, and most reliable dementia screening test is of great importance. Information presented in 2004 by one of us (PD) provided evidence that his Q & E test (see Chapter 4) was more sensitive than several other brief screening tests in detecting very mild dementia, but larger studies are needed.

Ideally, a blood or urine test for AD will become available, but the available candidates, such as the neural thread protein (see Chapter 4), have not gained widespread acceptance. Research in this area is ongoing. For example, a protein marker on blood platelets is under intense investigation.

Advances in Treatment

The good news on the treatment frontier is that many drugs are in the investigational phases. Unfortunately, many of them will not achieve FDA approval for several years. One of these new treatments is a vaccine for AD that was developed by Dale Schenck of Elan Pharmaceuticals. This vaccine includes the Aβ42 peptide and causes the body to produce antibodies directed against this peptide. The Aβ42 peptide encourages amyloid plaque formation. When the antibody attaches to the peptide, it signals the immune cells to destroy the amyloid. In preliminary tests with mice, vaccination resulted in the destruction of the plaques or, if given early enough, prevented plaque development. Unfortunately, when the vaccine was tested in humans, a small percentage of patients developed a severe brain inflammation that resulted in termination of the trial. Autopsies of these patients showed that the parts of the brain that were *not* involved in the inflammatory response had fewer plaques than expected, although there were still many neurofibrillary tangles present. In addition, the patients in the trial who produced the antibody as a result of the vaccine, but did not develop encephalitis, had less progression of AD than those who did not produce antibody. Consequently, the vaccine's manufacturers are testing a newer version of the vaccine, which they believe will minimize the risk of encephalitis while still preserving the antibody response to the Aβ42 peptide. It is anticipated that results from these trials will be available in 2006.

Other innovative approaches to the treatment of AD include: 1) the use of nerve growth factor; 2) stem cells; 3) chemicals that inhibit β or γ-secretase activity; and 4) drugs that enhance glutamate activity. Nerve growth factor, which is produced naturally in the body, promotes the growth and survival of nerve cells. Unfortunately, it cannot cross easily into the brain from the bloodstream. Initial testing using synthetic nerve growth factor involved its administration directly into the brain via a tube placed in the brain ventricles. More recently, genetically engineered cells (called *fibroblasts*) that live in connective tissue and produce nerve growth factor are being transplanted into the brain. If either of these procedures is successful, their use may be restricted by their invasive nature.

An important advance that illustrates how basic research can potentially influence treatment decisions was made by S. Oddo and his colleagues at UC Irvine. Using mice that had been genetically engineered to overproduce both amyloid and tau protein, they showed that a vaccine directed against amyloid cleared not only the amyloid protein, but if given early enough in the disease course, the tau protein as well. These results imply that if a vaccine does become clinically available, it will need to be given early to be maximally effective, again highlighting the importance of early diagnosis. These researchers found that timely administration of a γ-secretase inhibitor also resulted in the clearing of amyloid and tau deposits.

A medication called Alzhemed®, which interacts with amyloid fibrils, was found in preliminary clinical studies to be beneficial. Larger studies with this drug began in late 2004.

Ronald Reagan's death from Alzheimer's disease has brought the idea of stem cell research back into the national spotlight. Nancy and her son, Ron Reagan, have championed this type of research. The potential

> Ronald Reagan's death from Alzheimer's disease has brought the idea of stem cell research back into the national spotlight.

for embryonic stem cells to treat AD is unknown, but clearly much more research is needed in this area. As of this writing, the pace of stem cell research is being slowed by federal regulations that forbid federal funding of research on newly created embryonic stem cell lines, but this may change with future legislation.

The last two new possible treatments for AD that will be mentioned here involve the inhibition of an enzyme that may lead to pathologic substances in the brain, and the enhancement of a neurotransmitter that is necessary for learning and memory. New medications that interfere with amyloid formation by blocking β- or γ-secretase activity are in various stages of clinical testing. Medications that interact with the glutamate neurotransmitter system—such as *ampakines*, which stimulate the AMPA glutamate receptor—and second generation glutamate NMDA receptor blockers are under development.

Prevention of the progression of MCI to AD is a major focus of interest, and several trials are in progress using medications that are already available. Trials of some of the statin agents used for lowering cholesterol, such as atorvastatin and simvistatin, are in the late stages of clinical testing. The results of these trials are expected to be announced sometime in 2005 or 2006. As mentioned previously, results of trials of the cholinesterase inhibitors for MCI are also in the late stages. Preliminary results of a study using Aricept® in MCI patients were announced during the 9th International Conference on Alzheimer's Disease and Related Disorders by Dr. Ron Petersen of the Mayo Clinic. In this study, Aricept® delayed the progression from MCI to AD by about 6 months compared to placebo, although ultimately there was no difference in the proportion of patients converting to AD by 3 years into the study. In another study published in late 2004 by Dr. S. Salloway and colleagues, it was announced that patients with MCI who were treated with Aricept® showed improvement on some (but not all) measures of cognitive performance. It is important to note, however, that no medication is as yet approved by the FDA for the treatment of MCI, and the jury remains very much out as to just how effective the present AD medications are in treating this condition.

An area of research that is revolutionizing all of biology—and that may soon have therapeutic applications in AD and other dementias—involves molecules called *small interfering RNA*, or *siRNA*, for short. The traditional "central dogma" of molecular biology states that the genetic code, or DNA, directs the production of messenger RNA (mRNA), which in turn synthesizes proteins. siRNA adds an additional level of regulation by its ability to interfere selectively with mRNA. These recently discovered, but evolutionarily ancient, short stretches of RNA are present naturally in cells and can very specifically turn off the production of a given protein. Scientists are now making artificial siRNA molecules that are designed to inhibit targeted proteins. Already a synthetic siRNA directed against the APP protein has been made and is being tested in mice. siRNAs directed against the β- and γ-secretase enzymes are under study. There is great hope that this explosive area of research will have a profound impact on the medicine of the future, although it is still a long way from clinical use.

Another important focus of future research is the prevention of AD in the first place. As we discussed in the chapter on risk factors, a large number of behavioral and dietary factors have been implicated in influencing the risk of developing AD. For example, an article by M.C. Morris and colleagues published in August 2004 showed for the first time a lowered risk of AD in people with higher dietary intake of niacin. Perhaps adoption of a healthier lifestyle in the general population will lead to a decline in the rate of AD. In fact, Dr. Gary Small of UCLA has started a research program to investigate the effects of a 14-day memory and lifestyle training program on brain metabolism in the normal elderly. This program is described in his book *The Memory Prescription: Dr. Gary Small's 14-Day Plan to Keep Your Brain and Body Young*. In small pilot studies, he is already finding some differences in the PET scans of the participants in his program, although it is still far too early to say for sure that this or similar programs will actually work to prevent AD.

COMMUNITY SUPPORT

Research efforts can only be successful if individuals volunteer to help evaluate the effectiveness of new treatments. AD patients and their families can help with research in several ways:

- Patients may consider participating in a clinical trial for a new medication.
- Patients and caregivers may volunteer for investigations of the social and emotional experience of AD.
- AD patients, caregivers, or other interested persons may donate their brains to a brain bank for use in future scientific studies.

There are some important things to consider when deciding whether to volunteer for a drug trial. The trial will likely include a group of patients who receive placebo treatment (essentially no treatment) or standard medical care for AD, which may mean treatment with an older medication. Even if the patient does receive a new drug, there may be negative side effects, some potentially serious. If these risks are explained to the patient and he is willing to participate, then they may receive some benefits. If the medication being tested is effective, then the patient will be among the first to receive it when the trials are completed. Also, patients participating in clinical trials generally receive free doctor visits and tests connected with the study. Two Web sites that list ongoing trials are www.centerwatch.com, which as of March 2004, reports 187 ongoing trials for AD and 40 trials for dementia, and the Alzheimer's Association site, www.alz.org.

Patients and caregivers may also choose to participate in research where the patient's and family's experiences are monitored, but there is no intervention. For example, they may be asked to provide information about social and emotional issues, the quality of life of the patient and caregiver, or the cognitive status of the participants. There may be no treatment involved, or families may be instructed to simply follow their physician's orders.

Lastly, researchers can extract valuable information from the brains of Alzheimer's patients, as well as healthy adults. By donating their brains to be used for research after their death, people can contribute to new insights regarding the development and progression of an illness, effects of treatments on the brain, or the effects of normal aging. For information about brain donation, please consult the Web site: www.brainbank.mclean.org/Donate.html. The importance of brain donation on scientific research on the brain and Alzheimer's disease cannot be overstated.

A special concern regarding individuals suffering a progressive illness is whether they are able to give the appropriate consent. People whose decision-making abilities are incapacitated by disease cannot be enrolled in trials against their will, and the question of how well a dementia patient can actually weigh the risks and benefits of participating in a clinical trial is difficult to establish. In practice, the details of the experiment are explained to both the patient and caregiver, and both sign the consent forms if they wish to participate. Participation in research is a personal decision that should be considered with family and physician input. Those who choose to volunteer give an invaluable gift to all mankind.

CONCLUSION

Patients, caregivers, doctors and other healthcare professionals, scientists, research institutes, health care systems, and society in general all have critically important roles to play in finding ways to combat the terrible

> The ever-accelerating pace of research is truly exciting.

effects of Alzheimer's disease and other causes of dementia. The ever-accelerating pace of research into the basic disease mechanisms, diagnostic methods, and new treatments is truly exciting. We are hopeful that readers of this book will have gained a solid foundation in understanding what we know about dementia, and, hence, will be in a much better position to understand the significance of future developments.

Glossary

Aβ42: A toxic fragment of the amyloid precursor protein that is important in the Alzheimer's disease process.

Acetylcholine: A brain chemical important for learning and memory.

Acetylcholinesterase Inhibitors: Medications that block the action of acetylcholinesterase, an enzyme that breaks down acetylcholine, thus raising the amount of acetylcholine in the brain. Examples include Aricept®, Exelon®, and Reminyl®.

Activities of Daily Living (ADL): A set of functional activities, such as dressing, bathing, or the ability to handle finances.

Aggregate: Used in this book to describe a tendency of certain abnormal proteins to stick together.

Allele: One member of a gene or genes that exist at a certain spot on a chromosome (a strand of DNA that makes up our genetic code; humans have 21 chromosomes). For a given gene, one allele comes from each parent, except for genes on the Y chromosome in males, which come only from the father.

Amnestic MCI: A form of mild cognitive impairment characterized by short-term memory loss, but with preservation of all other cognitive functions.

Amygdala: A brain nucleus important in emotional reactions and memory, the amygdala is located near the hippocampus and is part of the limbic system.

Amyloid Plaque: One of the two major pathologic findings in patients with Alzheimer's; amyloid plaques consist of deposits of fragments of the amyloid protein, together with the debris of damaged nerve cell processes and other components. They are found outside the cell, as opposed to the neurofibrillary tangle, which is found inside the cell.

177

Amyloid Precursor Protein (APP): A normal protein found on the cell membrane, the APP breaks down in an abnormal fashion in Alzheimer's.

Anosagnosia: Lack of awareness of a disease process. Not uncommonly, for example, the AD patient may deny he has a memory problem if asked.

Anticholinergic: A drug that antagonizes the action of acetylcholine. These medicines may impair memory and should be generally avoided by Alzheimer's patients.

Antiemetic: Medication for nausea.

Antihistamine: A medication that antagonizes the activity of histamine, a brain neurotransmitter that is also secreted by inflammatory cells. These are commonly used in nonprescription cold and flu remedies and help to dry the skin and mucous membranes. Some have side effects that are anticholinergic.

Antioxidants: Substances that help slow the destructive aging process of cellular molecules; examples include vitamins E and C.

Antipsychotic: A medication used for treating symptoms of psychosis, such as hallucinations and delusions.

Apathy: Lack of interest in activities; lack of motivation.

Apolipoprotein E (ApoE): A protein used in cholesterol transport that is found in three genetically determined forms. The ApoE4 form is associated with an increased risk of AD.

Aricept® (donepezil): See acetylcholinesterase inhibitors.

Ascertainment Bias: Term used in research to refer to a problem in oproperly classifying people in a study. For example, in AD research, a more highly educated person is harder to diagnose with early dementia, leading to a possible ascertainment bias in concluding that the disease preferentially strikes less educated people.

Astroglia: Brain cells that play nutritional and metabolic roles.

Assisted-Living Dementia Care Facilities: Living facilities that include special features designed to fit the needs of the cognitively impaired.

Atherosclerosis: A disease process caused by the accumulation of fatty substances and cholesterol in the arteries, which can cause heart attack and stroke.

Atrophy: Shrinkage of the brain, for example, as seen in MRI scans or upon autopsy in dementia patients.

β-amyloid: A fragment of the APP protein when it is broken down by certain enzymes; β-amyloid has a key role in the Alzheimer's disease process.

Biomarker: A biological or chemical sign of disease. An example of a biomarker would be the elevation of prostate specific antigen seen in prostate cancer.

Butyrylcholinesterase: A type of cholinesterase enzyme that breaks down the neurotransmitter acetylcholine.

Capgras Syndrome: A type of delusion where a person believes a familiar person is an imposter.

Carpal Tunnel Syndrome: Pinched nerve in the wrist.

Cerebral Cortex: The outer surface of the brain.

Cerebral Vascular Accidents: Strokes.

Cerebrospinal Fluid (CSF): Special body fluid surrounding the brain and spinal cord; processes affecting the nervous system may be detected by changes in CSF composition or pressure.

Chlamydia Pneumoniae: Common bacterial infection.

Choroid Plexus: Special cells located in the ventricles that make CSF.

Cognitive Function: Memory, language, reasoning, etc.

Cognitive Reserve Hypothesis: Theory that highly educated people do better on cognitive testing because of skills learned during the course of their education.

Comportment: Behavior during social interactions.

Computed Tomography Scan (CT): Uses computerized x-rays to obtain images inside the body.

Conscious/Declarative memory: Memory for particular events (episodic memory) or facts (semantic memory).

Cortical Dementia: Dementia caused by a disease process of the cerebral cortex, as opposed to subcortical dementia, where the disease process is associated with damage to the deep nuclei underneath the cerebral cortex. AD is an example of a cortical dementia, whereas the dementia associated with Huntington's disease is an example of a subcortical dementia.

Creutzfeldt-Jakob disease: Rare, ordinarily rapidly progressive dementia syndrome caused by an abnormal protein termed a prion.

Delirium: An acute confusional state characterized by fluctuating attention, hallucinations, and behavioral symptoms. Delirium has many possible causes.

Deep White Matter Disease: Usually refers to small strokes in the white matter of the brain, which underlies the cerebral cortex.

Delusional Misidentification Syndrome: A person misidentifies relatives or other familiar persons.

Delusions: A fixed, false belief.

Dementia: Any brain disease that causes loss of intellectual abilities.

Dementia with Lewy Bodies (DLB) aka Lewy Body Dementia (LBD): A type of dementia characterized by the presence of Lewy bodies in the brain (seen under the microscope); DLB can be difficult to distinguish from Alzheimer's disease and may coexist with it.

Depressive Pseudodementia: Depression that closely resembles or is misdiagnosed as a dementia.

Diagnostic and Statistical Manual of Mental Disorders (DSM): Published by the American Psychiatric Association, the DSM is in its

180

fourth edition as of October 2004 (the DSM-IV); it consists of definitions of psychiatric and neurologic diseases that affect the mind.

Disinhibition: Diminished ability to inhibit socially inappropriate responses.

DNA Microarray Analysis: A recent research technique that is able to analyze multiple genes at the same time.

Do Not Resuscitate (DNR) Order: If a person stops breathing, or their heart stops in the hospital, typically a "Code Blue" is called, and hospital personnel rush to the bedside to try to resuscitate the patient. If there is a DNR or "no code" order, no action is taken and the patient is allowed to die.

Dopamine: A brain neurotransmitter important for motor function and the reward properties of experiences (e.g., whether you find the experience pleasurable or not). It is particularly deficient in Parkinson's disease.

Dorsomedial Nucleus: Part of the thalamus; another important structure for memory.

Durable Power of Attorney: A legal document that gives a person power to make decisions for another person.

Durable Power of Attorney for Health Care: A legal document that gives a person specific powers to make *only* health care decisions for another person.

Electroencephalogram (EEG): A common neurologic test that measures electrical activity in the brain

Encephalitis: Severe inflammation of the brain.

Encoding: Learning something to be remembered later.

Entorhinal Cortex: Part of the cerebral cortex involved with memory formation, it is located close to the hippocampus.

Epilepsy: Repeated seizures.

Episodic memory: Memory for specific life events.

Erythrocyte Sedimentation Rate (ESR): Tested for elevation in auto-immune diseases.

Exelon® (rivastigmine): See acetylcholinesterase inhibitors.

Fibroblasts: Cells that live in connective tissue; recently they have been genetically engineered to produce nerve growth factor and implanted into the brain as an attempt to treat AD.

Frontotemporal Dementia (FTD): A type of dementia characterized by personality changes and loss of social functioning; may be confused with Alzheimer's.

Gingko Biloba: A tree whose extract has been purported to help with a variety of ailments, including memory problems, poor circulation, and depression. Studies of gingko biloba with Alzheimer's patients have had mixed results thus far.

Glia: A variety of related brain cells that play a critical role in support of neurons; examples include astroglia, oligodendroglia, and microglia.

Glioblastoma: A generally fatal brain tumor.

Glucocorticoid Hormones: Released from the adrenal gland during stress; these hormones include cortisol, which have effects on the brain.

Glutamate: A neurotransmitter involved in cell metabolism; excessive amounts can be toxic to brain cells.

Gyrus/Gyri: The folds of the brain (gyri is the plural of gyrus).

Hemorrhagic stroke: A stroke characterized by bleeding into the brain.

Hippocampus: A part of the brain important for learning and memory; the hippocampus is found deep in the temporal lobes.

Homocysteine: A normal amino acid, elevated levels of which have been associated with the risk of stroke and dementia.

Homozygous: Two alleles of a gene that are the same, as opposed to heterozygous, where they are different.

Hopkins Verbal Learning Test: Verbal memory test.

Huperzine A: An extract from a Chinese moss that has been used to treat inflammation, fever, and memory loss; it is under investigation as a treatment for Alzheimer's disease.

Hydrocephalus: Enlargement of the brain's fluid system (CSF).

Hyperphosphorylated: Excessive phosphate groups attached to a protein; in this book, it refers specifically to changes in the tau protein.

Hypersomnia: Sleeping too much.

Hyperthyroidism: Overactive thyroid function.

Hypothyroidism: Low thyroid function.

Idiopathic: Disease of unknown origin.

Implicit memory: Memory for things learned subconsciously.

Insomnia: Inability to fall asleep.

Intellect: The capacity for knowledge, ability to think abstractly.

Ischemic stroke: The most common type of stroke; caused by blockage of a brain artery.

Isolated Amnestic Syndrome: A disorder characterized by severe short-term memory loss, but including preservation of other cognitive functions.

Kinases: A type of enzyme, involved in attaching phosphate groups to proteins.

Korsakoff's Psychosis: Amnestic syndrome associated with thiamine deficiency; mainly affects chronic alcoholics.

Lumbar Puncture: A neurologic procedure done by insertion of a needle into the lower back in order to withdraw cerebrospinal fluid for analysis.

Magnetic Resonance Imaging (MRI): A sophisticated imaging study; MRI shows the anatomy of the brain in great detail.

Meningioma: A generally benign type of brain tumor that, when large enough, can cause dementia symptoms.

Meta-analysis: An analysis of a number of individual research studies on the same topic.

Metastatic Cancer: Cancer that has spread from its original site of development to other parts of the body.

Microglia: Nerve cells involved in inflammatory reactions.

Microtubules: A molecular structure found inside the cell that helps to form part of the cell's "skeleton." It is important for transport of materials from one part of the cell to another. The tau protein helps microtubules to function properly.

Microvascular Infarcts: Tiny strokes caused by blockage of small arteries.

Mild Cognitive Impairment (MCI): Impairment of cognition in the elderly that is not severe enough to be labeled dementia.

Mini-Mental State Examination (MMSE): A standard test for dementia.

Multiple Cognitive Deficits: A subtype of mild cognitive impairment in which more than one element of cognition is impaired.

Myelin Sheath: Sheath around nerve fibers that helps them to conduct electricity.

Myoclonus: A sudden, jerky movement, often caused by a small seizure, characteristic of Creutzfeldt-Jakob disease, although it can be seen in advanced AD as well.

Namenda® (memantine): AD medicine that works by blocking glutamate receptors.

Narcotic: Painkillers that act by binding to the brain's opioid receptors; examples include morphine and hydrocodone.

Neural Thread Protein (NTP): Protein found in the brain; a urine test for this is under investigation for dementia.

Neurofibrillary Tangles (NFT): Along with amyloid plaques, NFT are a characteristic feature in the brains of AD patients. They consist of hyperphosphorylated tau proteins that are stuck together in the form of paired helical filaments. NFT are found inside the cell, in contrast to the amyloid plaque which is found outside the cell.

Neurons: Brain cells primarily responsible for communication in the nervous system.

Neurotransmitters: Specific chemicals used by brain cells to communicate with one another.

Nicotinic Receptor: A subtype of a receptor for acetylcholine that is stimulated by nicotine.

Nonamnestic Mild Cognitive Impairment: Mild cognitive impairment subtype characterized by preservation of memory, but impairment of other cognitive function.

Nonsteroidal Anti-inflammatory Agents (NSAIDs): A class of medicines that suppress the inflammatory response often seen in painful conditions. Examples include ibuprofen and naprosyn.

Normal Pressure Hydrocephalus (NPH): Brain disease characterized by impairment of cerebrospinal fluid flow, producing symptoms of dementia, urinary incontinence, and imbalance.

Oligodendroglia: Type of brain cell that wraps the neurons in a myelin sheath.

Oligomer: In this book, refers to a short chain or aggregation of the toxic amyloid protein fragment involved in AD.

Oxidation: A chemical reaction utilizing oxygen; it can release free radicals as a byproduct.

Paired Helical Filaments: Microscopic structures formed by hyperphosphorylated tau proteins that are stuck together; they are found inside the brain cells of Alzheimer's patients.

Parkinsonism: Symptoms similar to those seen in Parkinson's disease, such as tremor, stiffness, and slowness of movement.

Pathologic: Caused by disease.

Peptides: A small chain of amino acids, too short to be termed a protein.

Phonological/Rehearsal loop: A subcomponent of working memory used to keep a memory fresh or send it to long-term memory, such as repeating a phone number you have just been given in preparation for dialing.

Pick's Disease: A type of dementia affecting the frontal and temporal lobes and marked by personality changes and cognitive decline. Upon autopsy, the diagnosis of Pick's disease is confirmed by the presence of Pick bodies seen under the microscope. Pick's disease is a subtype of frontotemporal dementia.

Placebo Group: In a research study, people given the placebo, or "sugar pill" instead of the drug being investigated.

Polysomnogram: A test used for detecting sleep disorders. During this procedure, the patient stays overnight in a sleep laboratory for monitoring of EEG, heart rate, breathing, and numerous other parameters.

Positron Emission Tomography (PET): Sophisticated imaging test that looks at brain metabolic activity.

Practice Parameter: A guideline for diagnosis or treatment issued by an official organization, such as the practice parameters issued by the American Academy of Neurologists on a wide variety of neurologic topics, including dementia.

Presenile Dementia: Older term referring to dementia starting at a relatively young age, such as under 60.

Presenilins: Proteins intimately involved with the γ-secretase enzyme and amyloid formation.

Pressure Sores (decubitus ulcers): In bed-bound patients, such as in terminal dementia, prolonged pressure on the skin from not moving can cause it to abrade and subsequently become infected.

Primary Progressive Aphasia: A rare disease characterized by selective loss of language abilities.

Prion: A type of protein in the brain.

Progressive: As use in this book, the time course of an illness.

Progressive Aphasia: See Primary Progressive Aphasia.

Prospective Studies: Medical studies that gathers groups of people together and conducts ongoing studies into the future.

Receptors: Molecules usually found on the cell surface that bind neurotransmitters and subsequently give signals to the cell.

Reminyl® (galantamine): See acetylcholinesterase inhibitors. In December 2004, due to confusion of Reminyl® with a diabetic medicine, Amoryl®, the manufacturer of Reminyl® (Janssen Pharmaceuticals) agreed with the FDA to change the name of Reminyl®. The new name has not yet been announced.

REM Behavior Disorder: Disorder of dream sleep where the person essentially acts out their dreams. REM sleep disorder is caused by failure of the paralysis function that usually occurs during dream sleep.

Restless Legs Syndrome: Common sleep disorder characterized by an irresistible urge to move the legs while trying to go to sleep.

Retrospective Studies: Medical studies that review the records or reports about individuals from the past.

Risk Factor: Anything that increases the chances of getting a disease.

Secretase: Enzymes important in processing the amyloid precursor protein. There are three types important in Alzheimer's disease, the α-, β-, and γ-secretases.

Sedative/Anxiolytic: Medications, such as Valium®, that cause drowsiness or a decrease in anxiety levels.

Seizures: Sudden changes in behavior, such as jerking, twitching, or staring, caused by abnormal electrical discharges in the brain. There are several different kinds of seizures, such as the generalized and partial complex varieties.

Selective Serotonin Reuptake Inhibitors (SSRIs): A class of medications used for treating depression that increase the amount of serotonin available in the brain.

Semantic Memory: Memory for facts.

Senile Dementia: An older term that is essentially synonymous with Alzheimer's disease.

Serotonin: A neurotransmitter important for sleep, arousal, appetite, memory, mood, and temperature control. Low serotonin levels are associated with depression.

Serum Thyroid Stimulating Hormone (TSH): Test used to diagnose thyroid problems.

Short-Term Memory: Memory for very recent events or facts, usually one of the first areas to become impaired Alzheimer's.

Single Photon Emission Computed Tomography (SPECT): A type of imaging study that shows metabolic changes in the brain.

siRNA (Small Interfering RNA): Short stretches of RNA present naturally in cells that have recently been found to play major regulatory roles in gene expression. Synthetic siRNAs targeted to inhibit the production of proteins important in AD are just beginning to be investigated.

Sleep Apnea: Common disorder of sleep caused by obstruction of airflow; symptoms include loud snoring and daytime drowsiness; diagnosed with a polysomnogram.

Source Memory: Memory for where a specific fact was learned.

Stains, Including Golgi, Myelin, Congo Red and Silver: Brain tissue is stained with dye in order to identify possible pathology.

Strategic Infarct Dementia: Dementia caused by a small stroke in an important brain communication area.

Subcortical Nucleus: Refers to a number of collections of brain cells (nuclei) found underlying the cerebral cortex, examples include the amygdala, caudate, and putamen.

Subdural Hematoma: Blood clot that can compress the brain if large enough and cause dementia symptoms.

Sulcus/Sulci: The spaces in between the folds of the brain. (*Sulci* is the plural of *sulcus*.)

Sundowning: Worsening of dementia symptoms at night.

Synaptic Cleft: Tiny gap between neurons where the neurotransmitters are secreted and picked up.

Synaptic Reserve Hypothesis: This hypothesis claims that an educated person has more synapses in their brain than a less educated person.

Synapse: Connection between two neurons, including the synaptic cleft and the nerve endings on either side of it.

Systemic Lupus: An autoimmune disease that can include cognitive difficulties.

Tardive Dyskinesia: A movement disorder that includes constant movements of the mouth and tongue.

Tau Protein: A specific protein associated with the microtubules in the cells. In Alzheimer's and some other dementias, the tau protein becomes hyperphosphorylated, resulting in loss of function.

Temporal Cortex: A part of the brain that stores semantic information and is important for memory function.

Thalamus: A part of the brain that serves chiefly to relay impulses, especially sensory impulses, to and from the cerebral cortex.

Tricyclic Antidepressants: Older type of medicine used to treat depression; characterized by three-ring structures in its chemical formula; examples include amitriptyline and nortriptyline.

Vascular Dementia: Dementia caused by strokes; second most common type of dementia.

Ventricles: Cavities within the brain that are filled with cerebrospinal fluid.

Visuospatial Sketch Pad: A component of working memory that allows one to review a visualization of an object or area.

Waveforms: Patterns seen in neurodiagnostic brain tests of electrical activity, such as in the EEG.

Abbreviations

(Note some of these are described in further detail in the Glossary.)

α, β, γ—alpha, beta, and gamma, the first three letters of the Greek alphabet

AAMI—Age associated memory impairment

AAN—American Academy of Neurology

ACE—Addenbrooke's Cognitive Examination

AD—Alzheimer's disease

ADAS-cog—Alzheimer's Disease Assessment Scale—cognitive section

ADDL—Amyloid-beta Derived Diffusible Ligands

ADL—Activities of daily living

ALDC—Assisted living dementia care

ApoE—Apolipoprotein E

APP—Amyloid precursor protein

CBC—Complete blood count

CIBIC+—Clinician's interview-based impression of change (the plus sign means with caregiver input)

CIND—Cognitively impaired, not demented

CDR—Clinical Dementia Rating scale

CJD—Creutzfeldt-Jakob disease

CPR—Cardiopulmonary resuscitation

CSF—Cerebrospinal fluid

CT—Computed tomography

CVA—Cerebrovascular accident (stroke)

DNR—"Do Not Resuscitate" order

DSM—Diagnostic and Statistical Manual (of the American Psychiatric Association)

EEG—Electroencephalogram

FAQ—Functional Activities Questionnaire

FDA—Food and Drug Administration

FTD—Frontotemporal dementia

GDS—Global Deterioration Scale

GPS—Global Positioning Satellite

LBD—Lewy body dementia aka DLB (dementia with Lewy bodies)

LP—Lumbar puncture

MCI—Mild Cognitive Impairment

MMSE—Mini-Mental State Examination

MRI—Magnetic Resonance Imaging

NIH—National Institute of Health

NLDC—Nursing level dementia care

NPH—Normal Pressure Hydrocephalus

NSAID—Nonsteroidal Anti-inflammatory Drug

siRNA—Small interfering RNA

SSRI—Selective Serotonin Reuptake Inhibitor

PET—Positron Emission Tomography

REM—Rapid eye movement

SPECT—Single photon emission computerized tomography

NPI—Neuropsychiatric Inventory

NTP—Neuronal thread protein

RBANS—Repeatable Battery for Assessment of Neuropsychological Status

Q & E—Quick and Easy dementia screening test developed by Dr. Dash

Resources

INFORMATIVE WEB SITES

The Alzheimer's Association: www.alz.org

The National Council on Aging: www.ncoa.org

The National Family Caregivers Association: www.nfcacares.org

Alzheimer's Disease Education and Referral Center: www.alzheimers.org/adear (24-hour help line: 1-800-272-3900)

The Ribbon (on-line newsletter for caregivers): www.theribbon.com

The Eldercare Locator: http://www.eldercare.gov

The Safe Return Program: www.alz.org/Services/SafeReturn.asp

AD drug sites: www.aricept.com; www.reminyl.com; www.exelon.com; www.namenda.com

University of Florida AD site: www.alzon-line.com

Mayo Clinic (click on Alzheimer's center on the main site): www.mayoclinic.com

Scientific literature searches: www.pubmed.com

Genetic tests: http://www.genetests.org

Products to aid in an independent lifestyle: www.age-in-place.com

Safety tips: http://www.alzheimers-illinois.org/tips/safety.html

Medicare-approved nursing facilities: www.medicare.gov/Nursing/Overview.asp

Free referral services for nursing facilities: www.aplaceformom.com, or by calling 1-877-666-3239

Drug trials (ongoing): www.centerwatch.com (reports 187 ongoing trials for AD and 40 trials for dementia); also Alzheimer's Association site: www.alz.org

Brain donation: www.brainbank.mclean.org/Donate.html

PUBLICATIONS

The Complete Guide to Alzheimer's Proofing Your Home, by M.L. Warner.

The 36-Hour Day by Nancy Mace and Peter Rabins.

The Mayo Clinic on Alzheimer's Disease by Mayo Clinic.

Alzheimer's for Dummies by Patricia Smith, Mary Kenan, Mark Kunik, and Leeza Gibbons.

The Memory Prescription by Dr. Gary Small of UCLA (14-day memory and lifestyle training program).

Love is Ageless: Stories about Alzheimer's Disease. Edited by Jessica Bryan.

Index

preventing AD, 129–142
primary progressive aphasia, 70
prion diseases, 70
probable vs. possible AD diagnosis, 6
progressive nature of diseases, 2–3,
   51–52
Propranolol. *See* inderal
prospective research studies,
   129–131
Provera. *See* medroxyprogesterone
Prozac. *See* fluoxetine
Prusiner, Stanley, 70
pseudodementia and depression, 84
psychotic symptoms, treatment of,
   109–111

quetiapine (Seroquel), 110
Quick and Easy (Q&E) Dementia
   Screening Test, 39–40

rate of decline in AD, 51–52
Reagan, Ronald, 172
recall and memory, 26–27
receptors, in neurons, 31–32
refusal to seek diagnosis/treatment,
   54–55
rehearsal loop in memory, 26
REM behavior disorder, 113
Reminyl. *See* galantamine
Repeatable Battery for the
   Assessment of
   Neuropsychological Stauts
   (RBANS), 41
research into AD, 129–131, 167–176
   brain donation as, 175
   cause of AD and, 168–169
   community support for, 174–176
   diagnostic advances and,
      169–171
   microarray analysis in, 168–169
   participation in, 174–176
   treatment advances and, 171–174
restless legs syndrome, 112
retrospective research studies,
   129–131
reversible dementias, 57–65, 58t
risk factors for AD, 129–142, 131t,
   174

risk factors for AD *(continued)*
   age as, 132
   alcohol abuse as, 136–138
   aluminum intake and, 141
   cardiovascular risk factors and,
      135–136
   diet and, 134–135
   education and general
      intelligence as, 138–140
   ethnicity as, 132
   exercise and, 137–138
   genetics as, 132–134
   head injury as, 141
   hormones and, 140
   modifiable, 134–141
   nonmodifiable, 132–134
   smoking as, 136–138
   stress as, 140
risperidone (Risperdal), 110
rivastigmine (Exelon), 32, 91, 92t,
   95–96, 99, 102, 103, 109
RNA research, 173–174
rofecoxib (Vioxx), 126

safety considerations with AD,
   148–149
Scoville, William, 23–24
screening for AD/dementia, 16–19,
   18t, 37. *See also* bedside tests of
   mental status
   genetic testing and, 46, 132–134
secretase pathways (alpha, beta,
   gamma), 76–78, 171, 173–174
sedatives, 62
seizure disorders, 44, 117–118
*Selecting a Nursing Home with a
   Dedicated Dementia Unit*, 152
selective serotonin reuptake
   inhibitors (SSRIs), 108–109
semantic dementia, 31
semantic memory, 28
senile dementia, 1
sensorium and AD, 5
sensory memory, 24–26, **24**
Seroquel. *See* quetiapine
sertraline (Zoloft), 108, 115
sexual behavior, inappropriate,
   115–116